Yoga
American
Style

Yoga
American
Style

Prem Prakash

Yes International Publishers
Saint Paul, Minnesota

For information and permissions address:
Yes International Publishers
1317 Summit Avenue
Saint Paul, MN 55105-2602
www.yespublishers.com
651-645-6808

Library of Congress Cataloging-in-Publication Data

Prem Prakash, 1959-
Yoga American style / Prem Prakash.
    p. cm.
ISBN 978-0-936663-46-3
1. Yoga. I. Title
B132. Y6P675 2009
294.5'436—dc22

                              2009001835

Table of Contents

Yoga American Style

Turn your hand so your palm is facing towards you. Now spread your fingers wide. See the distance between the tip of your thumb and your pinky? That was about the size of the Philadelphia phone book when I was growing up there some thirty-five years ago. At that time, in that enormous metropolitan phone book, there was just one listing for yoga instruction.

Times certainly have changed. Everywhere you look there are yoga classes, yoga periodicals, yoga conferences, and yoga clothing and accessories. Yoga is being enjoyed by people who, not long ago, would have considered it the domain of fakirs and snake charmers. Yoga practices which were once the secrets of renunciate monks in secluded ashrams are openly shared in fitness centers, on college campuses, and in church basements. Yoga has become mainstream—an influential force in the fields of holistic health, stress reduction, transpersonal psychology, and interfaith dialogue.

Yoga has been in this country for only about one hundred years, and the transmission of this spiritual art from India is still taking place. American yoga will, and should, be different from the yoga of India. Of course, the essential teachings and practices must retain their integrity if they are to be effective. However, the manner in which the teachings are presented and how they unfold in our individual and collective Western lives, will vary greatly from that of our Indian brothers and sisters.

Many Westerners are under the false impression that the purpose of yoga is to become relaxed, free of stress, and better able to obtain their desires. While it is true that yoga practice does bring about a more untroubled attitude, to present this as the goal of yoga is to support a misperception that yoga practice is about becoming better adapted to the world. This takes yoga out of its spiritual context and diminishes the possibility of the radical re-orientation of consciousness necessary for realization of one's true nature.

Feeling good is fine and dandy, but spirituality, in the long run, is more about self-transcendence than about self-improve-ment. If yoga practices are presented outside of their spiritual con-text, they are no longer yoga. This is my criticism of most yoga classes given in health clubs and similar settings. The spa is a swell place for a swim and a workout, but it is an unlikely site for a spiritual experience. Can you imagine someone who claims to be a Catholic priest offering the sacrament of communion at the local YMCA because it is helpful in stress management?

Yoga in contemporary America is being advertised as a means to health, wealth, and comfort. As a result, beginning yoga stu-dents are sometimes shocked when they discover that yoga prac-tice reveals just how chaotic and disappointing are their lives. As a true spiritual discipline, yoga strips away the veneer of pompous self-satisfaction that we lay down to prevent ourselves from expe-riencing the depths of despair and longing that hide in our hearts. But it is only by first becoming aware of the inner turmoil which already exists that we gain an opportunity to fully relinquish the root causes of our suffering. When students come to me and tell me of the great pain in their lives, I am gladdened—not because of their pain but because they are the ones who have a real chance at growth. They have hit the wall, and they know that it is useless to lie to themselves any longer.

In his *Yoga Sutras*, Sri Patanjali defines yoga as the "stilling of the modifications of the mind." When the mind is stilled, what remains is consciousness untarnished, capable of reflecting the light of love. It is no more possible to attain this peaceful state without effort and upheaval than it is to build a house without labor. Relaxing and pretending that the house is already built just won't cut it when the cold winds blow. The construction crew has to get out there and sweat and toil to get the house completed.

Shankara has written that there are three great boons: a healthy human body, a desire for liberation, and an enlightened guru from whom one can receive instruction. It's easy to take the first boon for granted in our opulent society. Abundant food and comfortable living quarters make health more readily possible than most anywhere else in the world. The quest for the second boon, desire for liberation, is guaranteed us by the Bill of Rights through the right to religious freedom. This is a great blessing for us, as many people live in societies that severely curtail religious freedom.

As for the third boon, many in the West fail to understand one of the principal points of yoga: it is an initiatory practice. That means that one must, at some point, study with an authentic teacher. This may not mean much to one who has not undergone such a discipline. To those who have, the meaning is apparent. A good teacher can support and confront a student in a manner the student could never do on his own. A good teacher can push buttons that the student doesn't even know he has. The acceptance of a teacher is a necessary and vitally significant milestone on the path. One does not remain forever at a milestone, but neither does one reach his destination without passing it by.

How does one know an authentic teacher? In our marketplace society, anyone who takes out an ad in the yellow pages becomes a yoga teacher. But if you're willing to take your car to a guy who just thinks he's a competent mechanic . . . well, good luck! On the other hand, some yoga associations have formal training programs from which one graduates with a certificate or diploma, making one an "authentic" yoga teacher. I support their efforts because they at least weed out the frauds and incompetents. But becoming a yoga teacher is not the same as becoming competent in any other subject.

The techniques of some yoga practices, such as sitting properly, can be taught. However, practices are only significant to the extent that they support the attainment of Self-realization. And this realization is unlike any area of objective study. Enlightenment is about the one who does the studying, not about any body of knowledge. An authentic teacher is one who knows his Self and can help others come to the same wisdom.

My personal opinion is that one becomes a yoga teacher when his teacher gives him permission to teach. This is how transmission of spiritual authority is generated, and this is how the energy of teachers is passed down through a lineage. Competency is part of the equation, but neither Jesus nor the Buddha ever graduated from a training program. They both did, however, study with teachers prior to undertaking their teaching missions.

No one knows what American yoga will look like in the new millennium. At the present time, the seeds the great teachers from India planted in this country are still growing. You and I are the soil in which these seeds may eventually bear fruit. The transmission of the teachings from the land of Shiva and Ganesha to the home of Uncle Sam and Mickey Mouse is going to be very interesting. It offers us a great opportunity, but it also demands that we treat yoga with the respect it deserves.

The Branches of Yoga

There are several branches of yoga traditionally cited as valid approaches to the goal of Self-realization. Yoga, in its fullest sense, however, is not so much a tree with different branches as it is a comprehensive spiritual art that takes into account the varied needs of different individuals and even the same individual at different times. As Sri Krishna Prem so eloquently stated, "Yoga is not a synthesis of all the separate branches of the tradition; it is the prior and undivided whole of which the branches represent partial formations."

I would like to briefly explore the primary branches of yoga and point out their advantages and pitfalls. My hope is this will assist the seeker in understanding how yoga is a comprehensive art and science with many facets. The branches of yoga which I will discuss are jnana yoga, the yoga of wisdom; raja yoga, the yoga of meditation; hatha yoga, the yoga of physical processes; karma yoga, the yoga of service; and bhakti yoga, the yoga of devotion.

Jnana yoga is a path oriented toward realizing the eternal in its transcendent aspect. The emphasis of jnana yoga is on the discernment of pure awareness from nature and all temporal phenomena. The jnana yogi seeks to uncover his true Self, the *Atman,* in its state separate from body or mind. He believes that anything which undergoes change is not his Self and should be transcended. Shankara and Ramana Maharshi are two of the best-known exponents of this path, and the principal texts are the *Brahma Sutra* and some of the upanishads.

The *sadhana* (practice) of jnana yogi consists in the practice of applying the maxim *"neti, neti"* (not this, not this) to anything which is not eternal. By denying what is transient, he hopes to abide in the eternal. He seeks not so much to grow towards a spiritual goal, but to transcend all modifications of nature, that which has the potential for growth or decay.

The advantage of jnana yoga is that it provides a strong focus on the goal of Self-realization. Because the jnana yogi seeks the transcendent, he can remain detached from the emotional traumas, the physical problems, and the desire for the fruits of yoga practice (such as *siddhis*, psychic powers) that plague aspirants on other paths. The disadvantage of jnana yoga is that it can easily draw the aspirant into a deluded mental condition. It is easy for the inexperienced aspirant to confuse the elevated state of transcendence of body and mind with his own psychological condition of dissociation from body and personality. The former is a state of enlightenment; the latter is closer to autism. Immature jnana yogis often fail to recognize that God has two aspects: eternal stillness and eternal activity. By falling down on one side of the fence, by focusing solely on being, they fail to realize the joy of doing, the aspect of God in activity.

Raja yoga, literally "kingly yoga," is that branch of yoga which focuses primarily on meditation. The goal of raja yoga is the attainment of *samadhi*, a state of awareness accessible to the still, meditating practitioner. The raja yogi seeks to quiet all aspects of his body and mind and enter into a transcendent state beyond nature. Some schools define the highest samadhi as taking place when the breath has stopped, obviously necessitating that the body be in an immobile posture. Patanjali is generally recognized as the foremost exponent of raja yoga, and his *Yoga Sutras* are the primary text of this discipline.

The advantage of raja yoga is that it is a very precise system, which is accessible to anyone, regardless of current spiritual development. Raja yoga is a science, in which each stage of accomplishment brings an increasing degree of peace and wisdom. Any beginner can grab hold of the ladder of raja yoga and undertake practices which will eventually lead to the summit of samadhi. In addition, raja yoga has been so well explored that its system has been mapped very clearly, making it possible for the aspirant to work within a contextual framework in which he can understand his accomplishments and obstacles.

The disadvantage of raja yoga is that to truly climb its summit one would do well to live a rather isolated existence. Raja yoga requires great periods of time for meditation in a form which is best done in seclusion. It also demands extensive sadhanas for which the contemporary aspirant likely does not have the time.

Hatha yoga is a part of raja yoga. It is the branch of yoga that requires the aspirant to devote colossal amounts of time to physical processes, such as *pranayama* (breath and energy exercises) and *asanas* (physical exercises). Hatha yoga attempts to purify the nervous system and strengthen the body to such a degree that the hatha yogi attains a state of freedom from heat or cold, pain and pleasure, even hunger and thirst. Accomplished hatha yogis can remain without food or water for periods of time unreachable by the untrained human being. The hatha yoga tradition also claims that its adherents can attain great siddhis, such as the ability to walk on water or fly in the air. Two of the most renowned texts of this tradition are the *Hatha Yoga Pradipika* and the *Gerhanda Samhita*.

The advantage of hatha yoga practice is that it transforms the ordinary human body into a powerful vessel capable of great vitality and long life. In this way, the aspirant is not delayed in his sadhana by illness or physical discomfort. In addition, by extending the period of life the aspirant will, in theory, have enough time to complete his course of spiritual practice. Some schools even seek to create a physical, or super-physical, body capable of corporeal immortality.

The disadvantage of hatha yoga practice is, like raja yoga, a matter of quantity rather than quality. Hatha yoga can certainly bring a person to enlightenment, but its demands are unsuited to all but those who are ready to commit themselves to severe discipline. The true hatha yogi must live in isolation from ordinary society and undertake radical practices requiring fasting and potentially dangerous austerities. His sadhanas will take most of his day and night, leaving little time for other activities. If the hatha yoga tradition is still being practiced in its authentic form, it is taking place in remote regions of wild areas, inaccessible to the curious or mildly determined.

Karma yoga is the yoga of service to others and to God. It is a suitable orientation for those of an active nature, those who wish to work for the manifestation of the Kingdom of Heaven on Earth. The main thrust of the practice is the renunciation of fruits of action. That is, activities are undertaken for their own sake, the results being left to God. Activities are assumed for the benefit of the greater good, without concern for personal benefit. The path of karma yoga is described in detail in the Bhagavad Gita.

The advantage of karma yoga is that it transforms activity from selfish, goal-based action that results in binding karma, to selfless, ego-free action which produces no karma. In addition, karma yoga is suitable for everyone. As Sri Krishna points out in the Bhagavad Gita, no one is free from action for even a moment. Life in a body is based on action, and even the most reclusive hermit is constantly involved in some form of activity, no matter how subtle. The applicability of karma yoga for the busy modern person, whose responsibilities certainly exceed those of the hermit, is thus apparent.

The disadvantage of karma yoga is that it can quickly become a slippery slope of work-aholism in the guise of spiritual endeavor. The world is always going to need healing. If one were to work at service twenty-three hours a day, when he laid his head down to rest on the twenty-fourth hour there would still exist a multitude of uncompleted tasks and projects. Shankara's objection to karma yoga was that no amount of activity can produce spiritual growth because spiritual growth is the result of wisdom born of inner stillness. If this stillness is lost to an outer focus, regardless of good intentions, then karma yoga becomes a force of positive social action, but nothing more profound.

Bhakti yoga is the path of love and devotion. Traditionally, this has involved the use of external props and external relationships. Rites, rituals, and ceremonies comprise the props, and adoration of gurus and an external Supreme Being is the focus of the relationships. The beauty of bhakti yoga is that it is so accessible to anyone, regardless of spiritual development, because the aspirant is free to establish a relationship with God in any form that he finds attractive. In addition, it satisfies the primal craving inherent in the soul of all beings—the desire for love. Bhakti yoga satisfies this urge within a spiritual context, permitting love and devotion to be cultivated and directed in a healthy manner. The *Narada Bhakti Sutras* and portions of the Bhagavad Gita outline this path.

The disadvantage of bhakti yoga is that it can become an escape from the rigors of the deep self-examination required for spiritual growth. Devotion can all too easily deteriorate to a dreamy sentimentalism if it is not balanced with honest introspection. In addition, an overly emotional dependence on anything outside of oneself, regardless of how apparently "divine," prevents one from reaching the state of spiritual maturity. This has been the problem in those sects in which "grace" from the guru is supposed to be the fuel which drives the rocket of the disciples' growth. Gurus who claim to do the work the disciples must do for themselves are misleading their followers.

As we examine the different branches of yoga we can see how they each have their pluses and drawbacks. Too often, proponents of one system espouse propaganda about the superiority of their system, confusing aspirants. The wise aspirant will draw from the different approaches that which suits his temperament and personal life situation. In the same way that every individual has unique needs related to diet, sleep, and exercise, so does each have a unique spiritual path that is for his steps alone. It is my opinion that an aspirant should feel free to utilize whatever practices assist him in quieting his mind, opening his heart, and making him better able to serve others.

The World Is an Inkblot

A man goes to a psychiatrist, who decides to use a Rorschach Inkblot Test to evaluate his new patient. He shows the man a page with a large inkblot and asks the man to describe what he sees. The man tells the doctor he sees two people engaged in sex. The psychiatrist shows him another inkblot, and again the man sees sexual activity. On the third, fourth, fifth, and sixth inkblots, the man continues to see nothing but sex. Finally, the psychiatrist asks, "Sir, doesn't it seem strange that everything you see is erotic?" "What do you expect?" replies the man. "All you show me are dirty pictures."

A vitally important step on the spiritual path is taken when an individual accepts responsibility for his life and his experience of the world. Like our friend who sees eroticism in blots of ink, the external reality we perceive arises from the inner contents of our minds and the types of perceptions we desire. We are not passive spectators watching the world turn regardless of our wishes. Quite the contrary, we each live in a world of our own choosing; one which reflects our core beliefs, no matter how unconsciously held, about who we think we are. Formulating images of ourselves in our minds, we manifest scenarios which justify and support these images.

Projection is the great determiner of perception. Our inner world of mind, thoughts, and desires incites the dynamic of projection on two levels, the sensory and the psychological. On the sensory level, the world perceived by an individual is a mental phenomenon developed from the intercourse of senses and sense objects. As modern science tells us, all form is actually condensed energy, and energy is vibratory in nature.

When the vibrations of the external world strike the various senses, they produce the corresponding responses of sight, sound, taste, touch, and smell. The mind synthesizes these sensory experiences and produces a composite picture, which is then projected onto the external environment, creating the appearance of a world "out there." The apparently concrete, external world is actually a mental image projected onto abstract patterns of energy. This may sound shocking to our usual way of thinking, but it is entirely consistent with the teachings of the ancient sages of the East as well as contemporary physicists of the West.

On the psychological level, an individual projects his desires onto the sensory world, thereby creating his unique experience. That is why a group of people can drive through a town and each see something different. The hungry one sees the restaurants, the businessman sees the banks, the lusty one sees the attractive bodies. Each sees a town different from the others, based on his interests and desires.

One's psychological reality is also greatly influenced by projections of ownership. A man might own a coat and care for it with great attention, but after he gives it away he no longer cares what happens to it. The coat remains the same and its objective value does not change; the only thing that changes is the man's mind. He no longer projects onto the coat his desire for possession and the thought that it belongs to him.

What drives this mechanism of projection? In yoga, it is called *ahamkara* (ego). The term "ego" is used differently in yoga than it is by Freud and most schools of Western psychology. In yoga, ego is the part of consciousness which desires to identify itself as a distinct personality. It is the part of us that seeks to be different, to be special, to be better than others. This seeking creates a feeling of separation, and the ego experiences itself as apart, as opposed to a part, of life and of God.

The ego uses projection as a means of demarcating what it considers "me" from who it deems "other." In an attempt to rid itself of qualities with which it does not wish to be identified, the ego projects onto "other" people. People then appear as ugly, violent, cruel, and threatening. Projection, however, is a total process, and the ego's baby ends up getting thrown out with its bathwater. Those characteristics with which the ego would like to be identified, those qualities which it deems "me," also get projected. Different people then appear as beautiful, wise, powerful, spiritually advanced, and so on.

Projection inevitably results in conflict, for every ego is convinced that its projected values are right and proper. And it is the nature of the ego that it has little reluctance to attack, or even kill, when it feels justified. Thus we can understand the remarkable phenomenon in war that all parties are confident God is on their side.

Most people spend their lives trying to avoid pain by withdrawing from the "bad" things in the world and pursuing pleasure by obtaining the "good." But the ego is never able to quite get the world the way it desires, so frustration grows and peace becomes impossible. When a person psychologically projects, he gives power to the world to hurt him or to make him complete, preventing him from realizing the invulnerability and wholeness of Soul consciousness. No one can obtain what he really wants from the external world because what he really wants is inner peace. This can be achieved only when the dynamics of projection cease and the separative ego is transcended in Soul consciousness.

The decision to take responsibility for one's consciousness makes one a spiritual aspirant. The methods one uses to grow spiritually will vary based on inclination. What is universal to this process of growth, however, is that one becomes increasingly free of psychological projections and the resultant anger, jealousy, pride, guilt, and fear. With this freedom comes an increasing sense of the beauty of all life and the inherent sacredness of all beings. Assuming responsibility is the way beyond the ego, and the vision of the Soul awaits those who travel its path.

Purification

A man goes to a spiritual teacher and is given a small statue of a form of God. He thinks the statue is pretty snazzy, so he places it on the mantle in his living room. A few days later he notices how dusty the statue has gotten, so he cleans it off. While doing so, he notices that the entire mantle could use a good scrub. He cleans everything and is pleased at how well the shiny statue sits on the sparkling mantle.

A few more days go by and he observes that, compared to the cleanliness and simplicity of the mantle, the rest of the living room is quite the cluttered mess. So he cleans the living room and is again pleased. Then he sees that the living room is the only orderly room in the whole house. So he cleans the entire house, and again he is happy.

He's finally got his house neat and tidy, but now he becomes aware that his body is unhealthy and his mind is a chaotic mix of conflicting drives and desires. The poor fellow, he can hardly live with himself! His self-image of being a "together" guy, capable and cool, has given way to the recognition that his life was never under control. It's one thing to give the house a good spring cleaning, that only takes an afternoon; it's another thing to face up to the mountain of selfishness that lies buried beneath the superficial personality.

He goes back to the spiritual teacher and complains, "That statue you gave me must be cursed! My house may have been a bit messy, but my life was going fine. Since I got involved with you my life has gotten worse, not better. I'm ready to quit!"

The teacher gently chuckled, as he had heard this many times before, beginning when he said the same thing to his teacher. "My brother," he replied, "the turmoils you are facing are simply the initial results of bringing the fire of truth into your life. If you were not experiencing this upset, it would indicate that you are not sincerely applying yourself. When heat is placed under a pot of butter, the impurities rise to the top. Once the impurities are skimmed, what remains is pure. If you continue with your practices you will be able to skim the impurities of your ego and what will remain is your pure, golden consciousness."

When I started the Green Mountain School of Yoga in 1991, Baba Hari Dass gave me some instructions about teaching and what to expect from others. He said, "Many people will come, but if one in one hundred sticks with yoga practice, that is very good." That teaching has been very helpful because sometimes I could hardly believe that such promising students would, quite suddenly, drop yoga practice. I have had people tell me how grateful they were to have finally discovered yoga and they could hardly wait to participate in the next event of the Green Mountain School of Yoga. Then, I'd never see them again. I have since come to understand this as a reaction to the upsets produced by sincere yoga practice.

All of us carry a mental self-image of who we think we are. We live our lives based on this image and defending against what we feel threatens it. We're all idol worshippers, creating an image of ourselves and then adoring it. Our unhappiness arises when the world—in the form of sickness, disappointment, death—shatters the image we have of ourselves being a certain way. And since life is impermanent, no sooner do we get an image established than something comes along and destroys it. We generally respond to this destruction by quickly creating yet another image.

In yoga practice, an aspirant looks at his own mind objectively and watches it perform the function of image making. He sees how the mind establishes an identity for itself and how it constantly seeks to support and defend this image. Because the yogi can detach himself from the mind and view its operation objectively, he is able to extricate himself from its web.

At the final stage of this process, the aspirant will become aware that he is one with all beings. Before the aspirant can realize he is one with the saints and higher beings, however, he must first acknowledge he is one with those he finds less attractive. Before he can realize his consciousness is the abode of wisdom, compassion, and joy, he must see it is also the abode of selfishness, destruction, and murder. Before an aspirant can realize God lives in him, he must admit the devil also has a home in his mind.

The path through this chasm of fire is undertaken with two supports, says the great sage Patanjali in his *Yoga Sutras*. They are *abhyasah* (persistent practice) and *vairagyam* (dispassion). Persistent practice simply means doing one's *sadhana* (spiritual practices) every day. Some mornings it is exciting to jump out of bed and race to the meditation cushion. Other mornings it takes an act of giant will to slip out of the warm covers and sit facing the selfish, defensive mind. Practicing every day, however, is essential. In fact, during difficult times great progress is being made by arousing energy necessary to overcome resistance.

Spiritual growth is like an airplane trip; it is only in the beginning and the end that one is aware he is traveling. During a long portion of the spiritual journey one might feel that nothing is taking place. This is because the changes in consciousness are taking place on a level that is too subtle for one to observe about oneself. But regular sadhana will bear its fruit. If practice is carried out faithfully and correctly, it cannot fail to provide the desired result.

Dispassion, the second asset in the process of purification, means one does not become shaken by anything his consciousness contains. Dispassion is a two-edged sword. It means one should not become dismayed or guilty when he sees the depth of selfishness, violence, even perversity that lies within him. He is not to identify with these mental processes. Likewise, when he sees that within him lies the greatest courage, wisdom, or luminosity, he is not to identify with these aspects of mind. He is simply to watch them come and go. Consciousness, really, is nothing personal.

To discuss dispassion is one thing, but to experience it is another. Many yoga aspirants freak out when they begin to peer into their closet of consciousness and see the skeletons that hang there. To directly confront one's selfish tendencies can, at times, be overwhelming. But the only way out is through. Repeatedly, the yogi must adopt the position of the witness, silently observing mental phenomena without becoming involved with them. Thoughts are like rides at a carnival, each one promising some great adventure, a thrill or a chill. Rides are for children, however, not for mature spiritual aspirants who seek to know the true nature of the carnival and who is its creator.

When the aspirant first begins to practice dispassion, he may be astonished at how persistent thoughts are. Although his intention to quiet his mind may be earnest, still the train of thoughts keeps blowing its whistle. The great Tibetan yogi Milarepa faced a similar dilemma.

Milarepa retired to a secluded spot in the Himalayas to complete his search for enlightenment. When he sat for meditation in his solitary cave, demons appeared out of the thin air to disrupt his efforts. Milarepa was strong, and he determined he would fight the demons until they left the cave. No matter how fiercely he fought, though, the demons would not relinquish their habitation. Then Milarepa decided on a different strategy, he would ignore the demons. In spite of Milarepa's iron will, still the demons would not leave the cave.

Milarepa realized that fighting was not successful nor was ignoring the demons. Finally, in exasperation, Milarepa announced to the demons that he would no longer fight nor would he pretend that they weren't there. He just declared that no matter what they did, he would not cease his meditation practices. If they were that insistent, well, they would just all have to share the cave together. With that, the demons flew off.

Similarly, when distracting thoughts make their appearance during our meditations, it is futile to try to fight or ignore them. Both of these approaches only reinforce their presence. If one is quietly determined, however, one can take note of the distractions and then simply proceed with his practice. In this way, the temptation to pay attention to the distractions is overcome.

Through persistent practice and dispassion, the purification of consciousness takes place, and one becomes a vessel for great energies. Wisdom arises in the mind, and happiness abides in the heart. The way to enlightenment is through the fire of purification, which will likely sting a bit while the ego is being burned away. Remain confident, though, that the road to spiritual accomplishment is posted with a familiar sign: "Construction taking place: the inconvenience is temporary; the improvements are permanent." When purification is complete, the living God will rest on the mantle of our heart.

Who Created the World?

When I was a teenager, I held my first job, working for my father at his small auto parts store. Being exposed to the world of work and the occupations of different people somehow stirred me deeply. I became very appreciative that things do not appear out of thin air. Bridges, cars, offices, restaurants—these didn't just magically arise out of nowhere. Human beings had toiled for their construction. This may not sound like a bold realization, but it opened my eyes. I saw that what is created has a creator and that the former is brought into existence through the work of the latter. As a teenager I could only perceive this truth in the human realm; later I came to see that it is true in all realms.

The predominant religious belief of our time regarding creation tells of an omnipotent male God, residing in Heaven, who creates the Earth and all living creatures. The details of the story may vary a bit, but the basic structure is essentially the same. The presentation dictates an ontological reality in which one Being is the Creator, exclusively responsible for the whole of creation. All other sentient beings are the created, having nothing to do with the source of their world. There exists one Cause, who alone begets the universe.

The myth of the sole creator God carries in its wake a problem for the created beings. Since the world was created by someone other than themselves, they end up feeling like strangers in a strange land. In a world of immense complexities and little-understood phenomena, they must tread carefully perchance they violate some rule of order that could result in accident, disease, or death. The drama of creation may be divine, as says the Bible, or it may be a brutal struggle, as postulated by Darwin, but it certainly is as it is, regardless of the wishes of common folk like ourselves. Like an audience at a movie theater, we are powerless to change much of what takes place on the screen because the script was written by an ancient, omnipotent Other.

As an alternative to the story that the world was created by one omnipotent Creator acting alone, we may consider the yogic description of *lokas* (world systems). In this presentation, we find a vastly more complex and challenging perspective of the nature of creation, consciousness, matter, time, and space. In addition, we are told that creation is a constant process—eternity is now—and that our experience of life is in our own hands.

A loka is a collaborative creation of the sentient beings who share its reality. A loka is the creation of the collective consciousness of the beings who inhabit its domain and share in its perceptions. Like a spider who spins a web from her own being, so is a loka spun out of the consciousness of the beings who share a world system. Though a loka has a central creation point, the system itself continually evolves based on the energy exerted by the beings participating in that reality. Just as a city may be built and founded at one date but then change over time, likewise do lokas continue to evolve.

Each loka is a system unto itself, in the same way that ecosystems are fully complete. Lokas are also like ecosystems in that they vary greatly, just as the ecosystem of the ocean is vastly different from that of the desert. Some lokas are heavenly; these are the higher astral planes, in which great pleasures can be experienced for extensive periods of time. Other lokas are hellish; there the inhabitants experience much pain and suffering. And some lokas, such as the one which includes the planet Earth, provide a vast assortment of possible experiences. Here, some experiences approach the heavenly, some approach the hellish, and most are somewhat in-between—just right for a human being.

Imagine, if you will, a movie theater where the thoughts of each member of the audience can become projected onto the screen. In such a theater, each participant from the audience would project onto the screen what he would like to see. Some would be interested in comedy, others in adventure or romance, and some, as we know from the popularity of the genre, in violence and horror. In true democratic style, each member of the audience would have equal power over the creation of the movie. And, true to democracy, the majority would rule. If ninety people wanted to see a romance and ten wanted to see a tragedy, the movie would take the form of a romance touched with pathos.

With the creation of such a movie, the likely result would be each member of the audience identifying with what he created. Though each person creates autonomously, cooperation is possible in such examples as one person creating rain and another creating flowers or two friends finding one another. Conflict would arise when two people both want to be the monarch or win the same battle. We may ask why anyone would want to project any unhealthy personalities or painful experiences, but, as mentioned before, horror stories are very popular in our day and age.

Before continuing with the analogy, it is worth noting that advances in computer sciences and virtual reality technologies may soon make possible some sort of externalization of consciousness. A "theater of the minds" may well be a future form of entertainment or even result in the construction of some type of external, virtual environment. Contemplating this version of the dynamics of creation may help prepare us to serve in the manifestation of our future on this planet.

If the movie theater analogy is reflective of how creation operates, then we are responsible for the creation of our world and we are free to create the universe we desire. We could even say this is the intended use of free will. At the present time, we are creating our world under duress of an old religious myth, that of the sole Creator God.

The problem with this particular myth is that it perpetuates our sense of powerlessness over the past and the unpredictability of the future. In addition, the movie about Adam and Eve, and their original sin which condemns all human beings, horribly haunts our collective subconscious. We have been taught that sin, guilt, fear, and suffering are our lot and that we just might as well make the best of it. The materialist pursues whatever pleasures he may obtain before death ends his race. The religious man waits for his heavenly reward in the next life for the sufferings and humiliations of his terrestrial existence. Neither of these routes is satisfactory for the yogi. In Self-realization, the yogi becomes aware of the power and glory that are his by virtue of his divine status. He depends on neither man nor god, for his life is an expression of his own holy consciousness. He projects not scenarios of fear or dependency on the cosmic screen of the universe. He allows other sentient beings their free will to create dramas of pain and tragedy, but he takes no part in their production. Instead, he offers an alternative of peace and compassion: a beauty dream of love and healing.

Although it may seem impossible to imagine what a world without sin, guilt, and fear might look like, such a dream lies in the back of every person's mind, irrevocably planted there by the Divine. Many have become adult (as in adulterated) about the matter and have concluded that this beauty dream is simply some childish, innocent fantasy that can never be realized.

To the yogi, however, it is simply a question of responsibility. To accept responsibility means to accept that the world as we experience it is the result of our own consciousness. Everyone reaps (experiences in the outer world) just what he has sown (sought for in his own consciousness). The fact that the world seems beyond our control is simply reflective of the degree to which processes of the mind take place on a subconscious level. Through yoga practice, one makes conscious what is subconscious, where it can rationally be addressed.

Through regular spiritual practice, anyone can realize his true power. Such a realization brings with it a confidence in one's ability to regulate the flow of events in his life. As such, he can consciously participate in the manifestation of his loka. As a spiritual aspirant, he will naturally seek to manifest a world in which there is a predominance of love, harmony, and beauty. Cooperating with others of enlightened consciousness, we can celebrate that creation is in our own hands. Let us join with others and together utilize the power of our will to manifest a world without fear, a beauty dream of love and healing.

Grace

A man goes to a spiritual teacher who has a reputation for being able to perform miracles. The teacher tells the man that the miracles are irrelevant, what is important is the faith and devotion which makes miracles possible. As had happened so many times before, however, the man insists that his devotion can blossom only after a personal experience of the miraculous. So, the teacher writes something on a small piece of paper, folds it carefully, and tells the man to put it in his pocket. All this will enable the man to walk on water.

The man does as instructed and, sure enough, he strolls right on top of a lake. Amazed, he becomes curious as to what the teacher had written on the paper that could make this miracle possible. He pulls the paper out, unfolds it, and sees that written on it is the word "Rama," one of the Hindu names of God. He thinks to himself, "What's the big deal about Rama?" With this thought, he sinks beneath the water.

There is a long history of debate in theology about the nature of God and proper religious belief. The debate is rather irrelevant to yoga, though, because yoga is not about theory or belief—it is about experience. Once one begins to experience spiritual reality, the notion of entering into intellectual debate becomes absurd, like arguing over the hair on your head. If you want to find out if you have hair on your head, put your hand on your skull and find out for yourself. After that, it won't matter who argues with you. You will know the truth about the hair on your head.

The experience of spiritual reality grows out of the peace of one's own mind. This peace is cultivated by yoga practice: by detaching the mind from selfish thoughts and linking it with the power of the Divine. Although I like to refer to yoga as the science of spirituality, it is crucial to remember that yoga practice without devotion leaves yoga as just another dry, mechanistic system. Those who try to practice yoga without a spiritual intention usually get bored or burn out, because their egos are not getting sufficient attention. We may be able to put ourselves into convoluted yoga postures or sing devotional songs with a beautiful voice, but unless a spiritual longing lies behind our practice we are no different from gymnasts or parakeets.

Many Christians are suspicious about yoga as a valid spiritual path because they have been taught that one should not rely upon works to attain salvation; one should depend on the grace of God. This is a complicated issue, but one which can be clarified through the following three yogic principles. First, any condemnation of techniques which help people cultivate spiritual consciousness is man-made preaching, not God-made teaching. Spiritual practices do not negate the role of grace; they help cultivate one's sensitivity to grace.

Second, yoga does not see salvation, as the term is generally used, as a goal. We came from the One Self (which we may call God), and we live and move and have our being in that One. There is nothing to be saved from, except our own illusions about who we are and our relationship to God. Guilt and fear of God are creations of unhealthy human minds projecting their own anger and desire for vengeance. Guilt and fear are not only devastating to mental health, they have absolutely no role in spirituality. There is no God who wants to punish you.

The third principle is that grace is not some magical event, like winning the lottery, which magically blesses a few undeserving wretches, leaving the remaining wretches to suffer. Mother nature proceeds in an orderly fashion, and so does spiritual growth and experience. One depends on grace in the same way that one depends on wind to sail a boat. Before the boat is taken by the wind it must be hauled, lugged, and heaved into the water. Anyone who has ever pushed a boat into water from the shore knows how much work this can be. Still, there is a sweet moment when the water and wind take over, and one can hop on board and enjoy the ride.

This is also the way spiritual growth and experience come about. We purify our minds, open our hearts, and dedicate our lives to service. Yet these are only the processes of "pushing" ourselves into the spiritual waters. It is the grace of God blowing on the sails of our devotion that gives the ride. The great poet Kabir said, "I simply sit quietly, and God meditates on Himself in my mind."

The experience of God's grace comes to everyone in an individual way. What would we expect in a universe where we all have unique fingerprints and every snowflake is different? God arrives before us in a form that makes sense to us: as love or light, as compassion or joy, as a teacher or friend, as father or mother. It really doesn't matter how we relate to the Divine or what name we use as a label for this reality, which is far beyond labels anyway.

God is the ultimate shy lover: She will not agree to consummate our affair until She is certain we want nothing but Her. As long as the mind goes on repeating "I want . . . I need . . . I demand . . ." we will be stuck receiving the petty things we say we want, need, and demand. When we turn our mind from these ego thoughts and adopt the practice of focusing on God, then our Beloved feels assured that it is She we truly want. Our efforts then fulfill their purpose; our hearts open and are filled with the dance of God's love, twirling throughout our days and nights, bringing meaning and purpose to our life.

Why waste time trying to figure out how someone can walk on water simply by carrying God's name with him? It's much more fun to dance than it is to sit around debating music theory. Every day, let us push our boats to the water—by working on quieting our minds, opening our hearts, and serving others. One day our little boat will be close enough to water's edge that the winds of grace can billow the upturned sails and send us out beyond the shallows of worry and fear, out to the depths of love and life.

Taste the Mango

I once asked Baba Hari Dass, "Does the world exist outside of our minds?" I had been contemplating the relationship of the outside world to my inner environment, and I wondered just what was "out there" triggering the electrical activities of my brain.

"Yes," Babaji replied, the world does exist outside of one's mind. "But not in the way the mind thinks."

I inquired further, "Not in the way the mind thinks?"

He answered that the mind cannot think or perceive clearly. He wrote, "The world the mind sees is colored with likes and dislikes." He gave an example, "A man falls in love with a woman and thinks she is beautiful. Later he is angry with her and then she looks ugly. She was never beautiful or ugly, only in the man's mind."

"What does the world look like without the coloring of likes and dislikes?" I asked.

Babaji answered, "To find out what a mango tastes like you must taste it for yourself."

The practice of yoga helps one develop the ability to "taste the mango." Yoga clarifies the mind and nervous system so one's perceptions become increasingly pure and subtle, affording spiritual vision. The person without a clarified perceptual system sees his desires and attachments, his likes and dislikes, his problems and solutions, as being out in the world, outside of his own mind. He therefore feels powerless, at the mercy of external forces more potent than himself, which twist and turn regardless of his wishes or safety.

A traditional analogy used to portray our misperception of reality is that of the "rope and snake." We see a rope lying in a road and become frightened because it appears to be a coiled snake. We then run around endangered and confused as to how to deal with this ominous snake. The only solution to the problem of the snake is the realization that the snake does not exist. All the fear and confusion are solely the byproduct of a false perception. Nothing needs to be done about the snake; the solution lies within the one who perceives the snake.

Deep in our hearts we feel a nagging sense of self-doubt and dissatisfaction. We long for a way out of our fear and confusion, but we aren't sure where to turn. When someone comes along and tells us that our problems are based on misperceptions, we find some way to dismiss the message. After all, what could be more obvious than the danger that exists because of the snakes in our roads?

Anyone who is in a space to read this has arrived at a stage where, at the very least, he is beginning to question the conditioning he has received at the hands of the world. This conditioning reinforces the perception of snakes in the road and validates fear as a method for addressing the menace. A way of understanding spiritual practice is that it gives one the courage to ignore the screeching yelps of those who are frightened of snakes. Then one can proceed towards what lays on the road and, with clarified vision, decide for himself what is real.

There are some sure signs that we are misperceiving reality —anger, fear, confusion, and selfish desire. We can justify these in innumerable ways, but as long as we cling to the righteousness of our misperceptions we will not find any degree of peace. There are also clear indicators that we are perceiving reality. Two that I have come to consider benchmarks of right vision are compassion and a sense of humor.

Compassion arises from right vision because one finds it easy to empathize with those trapped in the terror of their own imagination. One who has become free of the pain of limping along life's path with a thorn in his foot will not run off to play once the thorn is removed. His desire becomes to see his brothers and sisters also free of pain. Once one's vision is healed and corrected, one only wishes to share this beautiful vision with others. The more who share in love's vision, the larger the number dancing in the ballroom of love.

As for a sense of humor, even a glimpse of the unreality of the snake affords one a profound giggle. What could be sillier than recognizing that we have been crying and complaining over something that was never there? What buffoons we have been, all for the purpose of protecting ourselves from a snake that never existed. Like a child experiencing a nightmare, we became so overwhelmed by our mental creations that we mistook them for reality. We forgot our spiritual identity and began to think of ourselves as mundane personalities under threat, requiring defenses against the world and others. How silly!

Let those of us who desire peace for ourselves and our planet accept responsibility for the world as we see it. None of us is perfect. As the Buddhists say, even the Buddha, in all his glory, is only halfway to the goal. Though we make mistakes, we retain the opportunity to clear our vision of illusory perceptions by purifying our minds and hearts. Then the dry crumbs of fear and anxiety which form our illusory daily bread may be transformed into a vision of divinity. This will allow us to taste, for ourselves, how delicious is the mango.

Karma

Much has been said about *karma,* and much has been misunderstood about karma, the universal law of cause and effect. Many presentations of karma make it sound as though it operates in a manner similar to the classic "billiard balls" example used to demonstrate cause and effect in Newtonian physics. There, ball a hits ball b, which hits ball c, which rebounds back into ball a. The example is attractive in its simplicity but does not reflect the subtle nature of karma.

Karma is actually not a matter of external phenomena. External events may serve as the manifestation of karma, but events themselves are effects, not causes. Cause lies within consciousness. The karmic initiative is rooted in the *vasanas* (tendencies) which reside in an individual's consciousness. Vasanas are the patterns by which thoughts, emotions, and behaviors manifest.

Every thought, word, or deed expressed by a person is a statement, be it consciously or unconsciously held, of how he wishes to be treated. By our thoughts, words, and actions we continuously create a subjective reality which validates our beliefs. A person who treats others with kindness and compassion is informing the universe that he desires to live in a world which offers kindness and compassion. A person who treats others malevolently demonstrates how he wishes to be treated. He makes a statement that he wants his reality to include pain and suffering.

All such statements of intention, both positive and negative, create a subtle energy pattern in the consciousness. These patterns are the vasanas and can be likened to irrigation ditches. When rain falls it follows the course of ditches which were previously dug. To change the course of irrigation, new ditches must be excavated.

Similarly, the energy of consciousness will continue to flow in established, conditioned patterns until new patterns are created.

Vasanas drive a person to manipulate his environment in order to fulfill the established energy pattern. This is karma in action; previously established patterns serve as causes for which present events are effects. The effects of the present events on consciousness then serve as causes for future effects, and so on turns the wheel of karma. Although this may sound like determinism, it actually provides answers for how an individual can gain control over his experience of life. Because our experiences are the result of our own vasanas, we can change our lives by changing our consciousness.

Though I say that we can gain control over experience, it is more precise to state that everyone already has this control. Because a sense of responsibility is incomplete, however, some domains feel beyond control. When we deny that cause lies in our consciousness, that we reap just what we have sown, then we feel vulnerable and frightened before the world. The greater the acceptance of responsibility, the greater the power over experience.

In discussions with spiritual aspirants about karma, two questions inevitably arise: "How did karma begin?" and "How can I get out of karmic bondage?" As for the first question, some of history's greatest spiritual teachers have refused to answer it! When asked, the Buddha did not respond at all, he maintained a "noble silence." The contemporary sage, Ramana Maharshi, responded to the nature of the questioner rather than the question. His answer was to ask the questioner, "Who is it that is asking the question?" The aspirant was to seek his own identity, and in the resolution of that quest all theoretical questions would be answered. *A Course In Miracles,* a modern synthesis of psychology and spirituality, answers by saying that pondering metaphysics is an example of "senseless musing." The answer to all spiritual questions is to be found in experience, not theology.

Having said that, it is this author's experience that contemporary Western aspirants often have a psychological need for some answers, even if they satisfy only the intellect. For many, a reasonable answer to the first question is necessary before they feel comfortable undertaking the practices that will answer the second. Let us, then, explore the origin of karma.

Since karma originates in the consciousness of an individual, as discussed in the first part of this essay, it is valuable to probe the relationship of individual consciousness and karma. As we do, we find that karma and individuality are mutually dependent, two sides of the same coin. The individual falsely believes himself to be a separate person who "has" thoughts, feelings, and ideas. In fact, though, the sense of individuality arises simultaneously with these mental phenomena, in the same way that a wave and a trough arise together.

For karma to occur, it takes "someone" to generate the karma. It takes an individual to produce a cause and later experience an effect. When no individual ego is present creating a cause, there exists no karmic reaction, for the chain of individuality which links cause and effect is broken. Phenomena—thoughts, words, and deeds—continue to occur, but these are realized to be unrelated to one's true Self. One sees that bodies, minds, and egos are part of Nature's process in the same way as flowers, rain, or thunder. The individual has no more substance than a fascinating image formed by clouds in the sky.

Although we may protest that without our individuality we would be faceless robots, the fact is that until we reach Soul consciousness we do not know what it really means to be a unique individual. Our egoic individuality is not much more than the result of biological and social conditioning. Pride in false individuality is like a prisoner bragging about his chains.

Transcending egoic identity is also the key to the answer to the second question, how to achieve liberation from the bonds of karma. At first glance, it appears the karmic cycle is endless and unbreakable. As we have seen, once a cause produces an effect, the effect then serves as a cause for a later effect, and so on, ad infinitum.

The resolution of this problem is to be had in the experience of grace. Grace is the descent of compassion from the spiritual realms. This divine energy helps the aspirant rise above the cycle of karma, an ascension which he could never achieve by his own efforts alone. Some of us have had the experience of trying to assist a trapped bird regain her freedom. When a bird accidentally flies inside a building, the poor creature flies every which way seeking an exit. She will often crash into windows and walls, perhaps even injuring herself in the process. When someone attempts to help her, she struggles even more, trying to escape from the very hands which can save her. It is only when she becomes exhausted that she finally becomes still and can be released outdoors, where she can again happily fly free.

Such is the manner in which liberation from karma takes place. When one begins to see that he will never be able to free himself of the karmic trap, he then humbly turns toward God and asks for help. This humility and prayerful attitude produce the stillness which enables God to "release" an aspirant from his egoic individuality into his natural environment of Soul consciousness, where he can happily "fly" free. Just as the bird is incapable of understanding how she is helped, likewise are we human beings incapable of understanding Who it is that helps us or in what manner the assistance is granted. Let us only be concerned with sincerely calling upon the Divine in whatever form makes sense to us and then simply be still and let grace descend. As the old adage goes, we should "Let go and let God."

Insight into the workings of karma helps one become aware

of the unity of all life. As one's consciousness becomes broad and deep, one can see how everything he does interacts with the entire universe. Like stones dropped on the surface of a still pond, one's thoughts, words, and deeds produce ripples in the ocean of the universe. As these ripples interact with each other, they produce an immense field of interpenetrating energy in which no part can be separated from the whole. This field is called Indra's Net. To touch one strand of the Net is to eventually touch all parts, for all parts are connected.

It is a beautiful fact of nature that positive change can be brought about in a much shorter time than it took to produce negative karma, just as a ditch can be filled in far less time than it took to dig. The divine structure of Indra's Net is such that negative ripples—such as selfishness and violence—are quite short-lived and have no significant results. Positive ripples—such as generosity and kindness—produce an energy which exists for substantial periods of time and generate long-lasting results. And love, being omnipotent and eternal, produces eternal results.

Freedom from karma is not brought about through fighting against karma, for struggle leaves one more entangled in the sticky web of cause and effect. Nor is freedom from karma brought about through some grand accomplishment, for all sense of gain or loss are of the ego. Freedom from karma is brought about through love. At home in Heaven, love visits the earth in the forms of compassion, service, and forgiveness. And only the light of love is warm enough to melt the icy chains of karma, leaving the Soul free of vasanas of ego, suffering, and limitation.

To be free of karma does not mean that one dies and receives some heavenly reward nor that one lives emotionally constipated, without inspiration for life or compassion for others. Just the opposite, by the alchemy of love, daily life with all its ordinary events and relationships becomes rich and fulfilling. The mundane is transformed into the magical. Everything becomes infused with meaning, and encounters with others become opportunities to rejoice in the power of love. Every thought, word, and deed become a part of the divine symphony of God's creation. Indra's Net is transformed from a spider web of karmic bondage into a cosmic harp on which is played the music of love, harmony, and beauty.

Sadhana

Tulsi Dass, best known as the author of the contemporary *Ramayana*, was a great believer in the potency of the practice of *japa* (repetition of one of the names of God) as a method of spiritual accomplishment. So great was his faith, it is said that he cured people of their diseases by praying and simply saying, "Rama." His son followed in his footsteps and also became an accomplished yogi through faith in the repetition of God's names. Once a group of lepers came to him and asked him to heal them of their disease. The son of Tulsi Dass prayed deeply and quietly said, "Rama, Rama." Lo and behold, the lepers were cured!

Some bystanders who witnessed this great miracle ran to Tulsi Dass and described the great deed his son had performed. Tulsi Dass did not, however, respond in the manner they expected. Rather than being proud, he hung his head and muttered, "After all my teaching, my son disgraces me." The astounded bystanders asked Tulsi Dass how, in what possible way, had his son failed him? Tulsi Dass replied, "Alas, my son's faith is so small that he found it necessary to repeat 'Rama' twice."

I suppose this is as good a place as any for a public confession. My disclosure is that for too many years I misunderstood the goal of yoga practice and paraded my accomplishments in sadhana as having some value. I could sit in the lotus pose until my knees went numb; I could go without sleep in order to chant kirtan; I could fast, grow my beard, shave my head, put strings up my nose and cloths down my throat. What a mighty yogi I tried to be! What a misguided fool I actually was.

Once I had the good fortune to meet Swami Brahmananda Saraswati (then still Dr. Ramamurti Mishra). In front of a group of several dozen people I asked a question which I thought to be earnest but that the teacher recognized as revealing my arrogance. He called me up to the front of the room and asked me if I could sit in the half-lotus posture. I did so, and he praised me. Then he asked if I could sit in the full lotus. I took this posture, trying to appear humble in front of the group, but actually feeling quite proud of my asana ability. Dr. Mishra then instructed me to grasp my hair, which I did. He then asked me to pull myself up off the ground. Obviously I was unable to do so, and his point regarding pride of accomplishment was well made!

There is a tendency among almost all aspirants to sometimes feel they are special because of their spiritual accomplishments. What we fail to realize is that pride and arrogance are fires which quickly burn down the barn where the harvests of our efforts are stored. True spiritual practice results in humility and the ability to love and serve. The only "perk" resulting from sadhana is the opportunity to love and serve more. Other rewards—fame, fortune, appreciation—remain within the boundaries of egoic desires.

Few of us have the ears to hear the profundity in the simple, timeless teachings that spiritual guides present in every age: quiet the mind, open the heart, serve others. We are convinced that we must travel to some remote ashram, where a bearded sage will whisper in our ears the closely guarded, nearly forgotten teachings that will forever remain secret to the uninitiated. Many of us spend years applying ourselves to dramatic practices and painful austerities. Eventually we realize, as said Jesus, that the Kingdom of God is revealed to the simple and pure of heart: to those who can love as he loved.

Sadhana is the practice of spiritual exercises for the purpose of undoing spiritual ignorance and learning how to express the Soul through the mind and body. Sadhana begins with an "s," which stands for "sometimes." That is, when one begins spiritual practice he starts with formal periods of sadhana set aside from ordinary activities. Time each day is spent in meditation, prayer, and the focusing of concentration on one's spiritual intention. With maturity, though, an aspirant comes to realize that sadhana ends with an "a," as in "always." Spiritual practice becomes a constant state throughout the day. Formal periods of practice may still be engaged in, but they have no sharp demarcation from other activities of daily life. Everything becomes an opportunity for expression of the Soul.

Many of us become confused in our sadhanas, making our spiritual practices into idols which end up replacing the very goal toward which the practices are intended to lead. We become obsessed with the raft and fail to let it go as we venture toward the farther shore. Imagine a man who wishes to plant a garden. He works mightily at digging the necessary irrigation system, tilling the soil, and planting the vegetables. He waters and fertilizes the vegetables, and they eventually develop into the fruits of his labors. Unfortunately, he becomes so enamored with the gardening itself that he fails to harvest the vegetables. Instead, he starts work on another plot of land and goes through the same process. And then, yet again, the vegetables go to waste. He becomes a gardener, but not a person who enjoys the garden's produce.

I hope you will be able to learn from some of my errors and avoid thinking yourself accomplished because you can exhibit something external. The real measuring stick of one's current spiritual state is simply this: can you extend love in this moment? It doesn't matter how loving you were yesterday or even an hour ago. It doesn't matter how long you sat in meditation or how deep was your samadhi. The issue is: are you loving now? For the only time love can be made real is now. Hence, love is the doorway in the temporal for the experience of the eternal. Love is the essence and purpose of sadhana. Without love, sadhana is an unharvested garden.

Authority

The first of the great yoga masters to publicly travel to the West was Swami Vivekananda, who came to America in 1893 at the invitation of the Congress of Religious Liberals. He had accepted an invitation to speak at the Parliament of World Religions being held in Chicago as part of the World's Fair. At the Congress, Swami Vivekananda was one of the last to speak, having been preceded by a multitude of theologians and clergy. When his turn came, he began his talk with these simple words, "My dear brothers and sisters . . . "

Before he could go on, the audience spontaneously responded with a standing ovation that continued for several minutes. Those in attendance reported the collective exhilaration that caused them to offer their sustained applause, even before hearing the Swami's lecture. Vivekananda's brief introduction was so potent because he recognized that those before him were, verily, his brothers and sisters. His words rang out with truth. He spoke as one with authority.

A little more than a century since then, we find ourselves living in a fictional world. We do not expect truth from our political leaders, we know advertisers lie about their products, the Hollywood stars we admire are actors, and we rightly sense that many of those in the public arena use their personal charisma to exploit others. It seems we cannot trust our government, our business leaders, or even the guy who fixes our car. Worst of all, few of us feel in our hearts that our religious leaders have had a direct experience of the reality of God and can provide us with the same opportunity.

The point is not that the world is filled with terrible liars. The point is simply that we have come to accept falsity as a norm, and this has dulled our ability to recognize authentic authority. Exaggeration and game playing have probably always been parts of the human experience of business, politics, and flirtation, but they have no place in spirituality.

The slick purveyors of religions promising easy access to heaven or the threat of eternal damnation have left many intelligent people turned off to the entire realm of spirituality. But just as counterfeit gold implies the existence of the real thing, likewise do religious hucksters exist as the shadow of valid paths to genuine religious experience. It is important that we not use the prevalence of phony teachers as an excuse to avoid the work we must do to grow spiritually.

In the epic myth, the *Ramayana,* there is an apt parable regarding authority. Princess Sita had been kidnapped by the evil Ravana, and she was held captive in a grove near his palace. Her husband, Prince Rama, had sent his emissary, the wise and faithful monkey Hanuman, to search for his missing wife. Hanuman eventually found Sita and told her that he had been sent by her loving husband, who will soon rescue her.

Sita, however, had doubts about Hanuman's true identity. After all, she thought, he could be one of Ravana's evil partners, disguised and lying. Hanuman, as if sensing her distrust, showed Sita a ring he possessed, which was a symbol of authenticity and power given him by Rama. Sita was overjoyed to realize that Hanuman was truly a friend who could be counted on and that she had not been forsaken but was soon to be reunited with her beloved.

Symbolically, Rama is God and Hanuman is the spiritual teacher. We are all Sitas, individual souls, isolated and pressured by the wicked Ravana, our egos. Yet in spite of this repression, we still long for reunion with our beloved, God. We learn of the reality of God's love from one "possessing the ring of Rama," one whose personal experience grants authority. At first we doubt, but little by little we come to trust in the teacher and teachings, and all worldly difficulties dissolve in the light of our own direct spiritual experiences. We practice spiritual disciplines while patiently waiting for reunion with our beloved; the mystical marriage of the individual soul with God, the one Self. This is the cosmic romance of which the mystics speak, and the apex of the human experience.

Many of us in the West have taken the notion of autonomy to an unhealthy extreme, denying our need for a teacher, an accomplished authority. The spiritual path is such a razor's edge and the ego such a subtle phenomenon that it is impossible for ordinary people like ourselves to attain Self-realization without the instruction, inspiration, and grace of a teacher. As far as I am concerned, the likelihood of anyone I have ever met achieving realization without a teacher is about the same as their beating Michael Jordan in a game of one-on-one. I suppose they could get very lucky and beat Mike, but any gambler would be happy to wager against them.

It is wonderful to learn that spiritual truth exists and there are honest people who will share it with us. These beings live for that purpose only, to bring the perennial wisdom to suffering human beings. To come into the presence of such a being is the greatest possible blessing. If you are fortunate enough to have come to an authentic teacher, regardless of particular tradition or sect, I encourage you to drink at the fountain of their wisdom and apply their teachings to your life. If you achieve the purpose of their instruction, you too will become a person with spiritual authority, born out of your own direct experience.

Stages of Spiritual Development

In this essay I would like to outline five stages along the spiritual path. These are intended to serve as a contextual map which I hope can help the aspirant make sense of the major issues he will face in his spiritual growth. In writing this, I risk exacerbating a common problem—the tendency of immature aspirants to judge their progress, and that of others, as though they were engaged in some athletic competition in which the goal is to cross the finish line as quickly as possible, and certainly before the other guy.

This competitive attitude, rooted in the ego's desire for separation and status, is blind to two major aspects of the entire spiritual journey. First, spiritual evolution takes place within Nature's manifestation and, therefore, proceeds at a pace in harmony with Nature herself. This organic process skips no steps, so advancement on the spiritual path is, in some ways, like physical maturation. It is not better to be thirty years old than it is fifteen, though the older person will hopefully be addressing a more subtle set of life issues.

Second, the spiritual journey is entirely comprehensive. The journey begins with unity and ends with unity. The separate entity who wishes to advance beyond others is only delaying his own re-unification with them. All consciousness is traveling through the cosmos as one. The individual entities are like waves on the same ocean. Large waves have more power than tiny waves, but their "superiority" is only on the surface. Both great and small are part of one magnificent body that ebbs and flows as one.

Stage 1: *Shanti*

The first noble truth of the Buddha is *sarvam duhkam* (all is suffering). Some Buddhists say this means that the world is like a house on fire, within which we play like little children, unaware of our true situation. The house is our ego, our self-centered, separative identity. Like Midas, with his powerful but horrible touch, our ego-based identity brings suffering to every sphere of life that it contacts. Though this may sound drastic, the realization of the pervasiveness of suffering throughout the manifest universe is an important stage in spiritual growth.

For many Westerners, to say that all is suffering may sound somewhat pessimistic. We think this is how the world must look to somebody in a third-world country surrounded by poverty, starvation, and lack of high definition television. But if we turn the coin around, we can see that our wealth and leisure actually keep us from probing the depth of the human condition. We are so busy with superficialities that we never glimpse below the tip of the iceberg of our small anxieties and worries, beneath which lay mammoth fears and terrors. The pleasures, entertainments, and distractions that our abundance permits can be seen as endless avoidance activities. For if we ever sat still, in silence, that creature from the depths of darkness that we so fear may have a chance to rise up and devour us.

When we do probe beneath the surface of superficial life, we find that the only thing worse than not getting what you want is getting what you want. In the end all selfish desires are but seeds of discontent. They sprout roots of separative consciousness and branches of competition. They flower in pride and produce the fruit of disappointment, within which are more seeds of discontent. The realization that all ego-based desire results in suffering brings forth the search for its opposite, *shanti* (peace). This longing for peace is the wisdom which begins to untangle the knot of ego.

Stage 2: *Shakti*

In the quest for peace, the aspirant comes to the recognition that he will need great energy to accomplish all his life tasks without being overwhelmed and stressed-out. The aspirant is drawn to sadhanas which will improve his health and stabilize his emotions and mental framework. Experiments with diet, sleep, lifestyle, and various formal practices—such as *pranayama* (breath and energy work) and *asana* (yoga postures)—come into play in the pursuit of *shakti* (energy).

During the search for shakti, one undergoes processes of purification. To maintain a state of high energy, the aspirant realizes that his body, emotions, and mind need to be pure and strong. The ordinary person is like a low-wattage light bulb: channel too much electricity through the medium, and the bulb will burn out. The aspirant seeks to make himself capable of holding high levels of shakti, that he might enjoy the divine luminance.

Purity of body means that the essentials of daily life must be met in a balanced manner. The Ayurvedic medical system, sister science to yoga, states that there are three pillars of life: food, sex, and sleep. Food for an aspirant must be nourishing, fresh, and appropriate to season and his lifestyle. A vegetarian diet is extremely helpful for many reasons, though one should not become fanatical about any aspect of diet. After all, it is only fuel for the physical vehicle; it should not become a means of distraction from the goal itself.

Sleep should be taken in moderation. One should sleep neither too much nor too little. As the body becomes healthy, less sleep is needed because the body is not stressed and wasting the energy it obtained through food, water, air, and sunshine.

Sex, an activity that gives rise to great confusion and one too complicated to discuss in detail here, is not inherently a barrier to spiritual growth. Sexual activity, within the context of a consensual, mindful relationship, can be an avenue for the maturation of the personality and the satisfaction of the emotions. Sexual behavior, like eating and sleeping, is an issue of exercising moderation and using common sense.

Purity of the emotions and mind means that one must learn to remain positive and upbeat. One should look for the noble in all people and God's will in all situations. One must cultivate attitudes of friendship and compassion toward all other beings. One must serve as an example of positive energy for those who are dispirited. This is not to imply that life is to be seen through rose-colored glasses. The aspirant should, however, strive to serve as a beacon of happiness in the night of depression and despair in which ego-based persons live. Being happy is among the greatest services one can provide for his brothers and sisters.

Stage 3: *Ramlila*

As shakti develops, one feels himself powerful and confident. Life loses its burdensome nature and becomes worthwhile. The insight arises that one's small life is in harmony with the great tides of God's creation. And since God's nature is joy, likewise does one begin to experience joy in his own life.

Spiritual exercises which were previously undertaken in an effort to obtain a goal, such as gaining shanti or shakti, are now done simply because they are enjoyable. At the early stages of sadhana, one feels like a child forced to do homework when he would rather play. The alarm clock rings in the morning, and the beginning yogi wishes for nothing more than to roll over and go back to sleep. He does not understand why his teacher requires daily practice. He would prefer his sleep or coffee and newspaper to his morning sadhana.

Just as the child would rather play games than study, so would the immature yogi favor goofing off to undertaking his practices. Later, however, like a student who has matured and become an enthusiastic scholar, the aspirant looks forward to those periods when he can focus on his spiritual practices. He no longer performs them because he seeks something further down his path, but because he finds gratification in his sadhana. Like an artist who enjoys painting or an athlete who delights in exercise, the yogi relishes the opportunity to express his creative life force through his sadhana. This is known as *Ramlila* (the play of God).

Stage 4: *Lankabhayankaram*

With the acquisition of the vision of Ramlila, one might feel that his journey has reached completion. But this stage is only the prelude to full accomplishment. First, great obstacles which prevent permanent abidance in the sacred inner space must be overcome. From the very depths of the *chitta* (personal consciousness) arise fears, doubts, and defenses which are like a mighty wall obstructing further progress. In psychological terms, we might say that this is the appearance of the darker aspects of the subconscious which are resistant to change. They seek to remain the dominant forces in one's psyche, reluctant to surrender before the tendencies of peace and harmony.

This insight has been presented mythologically in the tales of Christ being tempted in the desert and of Buddha being tempted and attacked by Mara as he sat under the bodhi tree. In both cases the aspirant was victorious. Jesus put Satan behind him and went on to fulfill his mission. The Buddha persisted in his meditation until the forces of Mara were depleted, and he attained his supreme enlightenment dedicated to the welfare of all beings.

The term "Lankabhayankaram" is an epithet given to Hanuman, one of the heroes of the great Indian epic, the Ramayana. It literally means "terrifier of Lanka," as Hanuman is depicted as the destroyer of Lanka, the stronghold of demons. Hanuman is able to recognize a demon, no matter how subtle his disguise, and he holds nothing back in his battle to destroy the negative forces. Symbolically, Hanuman (the accomplished aspirant) is able to recognize the demons (negative thoughts and feelings) which might present themselves to his consciousness, no matter how disguised (attractive, distracting, or logical) they might be. With his mighty club (the power of his own devotion) he destroys their presence in Lanka (in his heart).

Each aspirant must eventually find that fiery part of himself symbolized by Hanuman—selfless server and noble warrior. The spiritual path is not for the meek or those who give lip service to some amorphous, untested virtue described as "non-violence." Gentleness towards others is always to be demonstrated, but one must be a mighty conqueror of the Lanka within. The demons of selfish desire and laziness will not surrender without a fight. They must be slain with the sword of vitality and enthusiasm for the battle!

Stage 5. *Ma*

The primal human sound, ma, universal throughout virtually every tongue, holds special significance in the yogic tradition. "Ma," in Sanskrit, refers to the Great Goddess, the Divine Mother, the Alpha and Omega of existence. It is She who remains ever transcendent, yet permeates every atom of existence with Her loving presence. From Her, the One Absolute, arise the multitude of relative beings. She gives them birth, and She nurtures their lives in the form of Mother Nature. She beguiles them with her veil of spiritual illusion, causing them to forget their divine status, while She also provides the props and supports they will need to become free of the illusion.

She laughs in divine intoxication at the blissful paradox of Her game. She is the peace that surpasses understanding because she lives always beyond the known. She is never bound by any human concept or idea. In India, She is depicted as Kali, the dancing, black Goddess with a garland of human heads hung on her chest, which symbolizes that all people will be called to offer their heads (egos) to Her. They can do so lovingly, in devotion, after which they rise from their beheading reborn as Children of God. Or, if ignorance and pride prevent them from humbly submitting themselves to this process, Kali ends up with their heads anyway through the defeats that life heaves upon the egoic man—ending with the supreme defeat, the humiliation of death.

Yoga is a rational system of steps that lead to this fifth stage, the trans-rational leap of faith into that which can never be known, only loved. Depicting this Transcendent as Goddess is very appropriate for our time, for we have become estranged from nature and the feminine values of sympathy, tenderness, and appreciation for the cyclical nature of life. Our rocket ships, our computers, and our atom bombs prove our ability to construct devices that demonstrate our cleverness at applying reason and manipulating Aristotelian logic. Great as these achievements might be, they leave us empty in heart, for the heart is the realm of intuition. Like Adam and Eve, we have tasted the fruits of our knowing, only to find how bitter is the cost.

I am not proposing that we abandon reason, only that it be informed by intuition. For unless we are able, when necessary, to leap from the knowing, defensive mind into the innocent, intuitive heart, our earthly accomplishments are nothing but dust. And, as our weapons of destruction suggest, we may end as dust if we don't heed the voice of this inner Goddess. Bedecked with Her garland of severed heads, She appears dark and frightening only because she lives in the shadows of our unconscious. As one progresses through the stages of spiritual growth, one comes to know that fear of Her is nothing more than a self-perpetuating illusion based on ignorance.

Aspirant, fear nothing! Doubt your doubts, be angry with your anger, and penetrate through the darkness of terror-induced nightmares to the bliss-soaked dance of divine life: born, sustained, then destroyed by Ma.

Of Kali, Swami Vivekananda wrote,

> Dancing mad with joy,
> Come, Mother. Come!
> For terror is Thy name,
> Death is in Thy breath,
> And every shaking step
> Destroys a world for e'er.
> Thou "Time," the All-Destroyer!
> Come, O Mother. Come!
>
> Who dares misery love,
> And hug the form of Death,
> Dance in destruction's dance,
> To him the Mother comes.

Royalty

There once was a prince who, being the son of a wise and powerful king, was also wise and powerful. One fine day he went to the river to take his morning bath. He felt so good that he decided to swim clear across to the other shore. He took off his royal robes and plunged into the refreshing waters. In a few minutes he was climbing out on the bank of the other side, feeling wonderful. Then, suddenly, he slipped on a rock and fell hard, banging his head. He lay unconscious for some time, and when he awoke he had amnesia. He could not remember who he was or where he was. He stood naked and alone, confused to the core of his being.

The prince found an old cloak along the river, so he dressed himself and walked to the nearest town. By his clothing, the people took him to be a common laborer. A local farmer took him on as a hired hand. As time went on, the prince became accustomed to life with the people in the town. The farmer adopted him as a son, so he had a name. He married a local girl and had children with her, so he had a family. He learned the trade of farming, so he had an occupation. As such, he knew who he was, where he was, and what he should be doing.

Years later, one of the king's ministers was traveling when he came upon the prince, now living as a farmer. He told the prince about his true identity and his real name, but the "farmer" refused to accept what he was hearing. He found it impossible to believe that he was, in actuality, from a royal lineage, heir to a throne. The minister's description of the wealth and power available to him sounded like some grand fable. As he was very busy with his chores, he found it necessary to send away this foolish man who prattled on about his being a prince.

The most frequently asked theological question may well be: from where does suffering arise? Many spiritual traditions postulate reasons based on their metaphysical premises. Thus comes the enormous variety of theories: misery comes from a fallen world, evil is from the devil, pain is God's test, and other variations on the theme that an external agent is behind one's suffering. The profound yogic tradition, however, does not attribute suffering to any external cause. Yoga philosophy holds that the cause of suffering is due to the unhealthy use of one's own mind.

If the great yogis are right and suffering is due to the unhealthy use of our minds, it then follows that we can reduce suffering by bringing our minds to good health. We do this, first and foremost, by taking responsibility for our own consciousness. We do not blame others, nor circumstances, for the suffering we experience. Honestly and truthfully we must search our hearts and recognize that the harvest we reap has indeed sprung from the seeds we have sown. If we imagine it has come from anywhere else, we are simply avoiding responsibility. In this way, we can release the habit of blame and actually change our consciousness.

The process of changing one's consciousness is undertaken with the help of the great inquiry, the *atma-vichara* (Who am I?). By searching deeply inside for the answer, we discover that all our social roles are temporary identities we have adopted. The forgetful prince came to believe he was simply a son, a husband, a farmer. In a sense he was all these. But, if he truly knew himself, he would understand that he was also very much more. To become a prince and enjoy the privileges that were his, he did not need to accomplish or gain anything, he needed only to remember his true identity.

All of us suffer from a cosmic amnesia, which in yoga is called *avidya* (lack of wisdom). We have forgotten the royal source from which we were created, instead believing we are our bodies. Our suffering does not so much arise from these bodies but the self-images they tend to generate, images that distort our true magnificence. Our work is not to denigrate our bodies; our work is to elevate the bodily aspects of life so they become sacred.

Until the prince remembers he is the son of a king, he will not have access to the resources that his father can provide. He will have to struggle through mundane life like a mundane personality. Until we awaken to the divinity that lies within us, we will not have access to the energy, the peace, and the love that belong to us. We will have to struggle and weep over the affairs of the world, from which we all, in our own ways, suffer. Like the prince, we need not achieve or attain anything in order to claim our riches; we need only realize the spiritual answer to the inquiry, "Who am I?"

The great sages of every spiritual tradition have come to us with one great, universal message: awaken and know your real Self. The pangs of suffering we experience in our daily lives are reflections of the deep, primal pain resulting from the belief that we are separate from God. In one of the gnostic gospels, Jesus descends into hell in order to free the inmates there. Yet no one would leave with him. It was not because they doubted he was their savior but because they refused to acknowledge they were in hell. Let us acknowledge that our unenlightened condition is hell and we want out.

The sun of spiritual practice evaporates the clouds of avidya. The sticky entanglements of the complex world wash away, and we stand pure and free. The burden of false self-images falls from our shoulders, and we access the peace and power which had lain dormant in our hearts. The darkness of confusion and suffering disappear before the light of spiritual intelligence. We awaken and we know who we are, where we are, and what we are doing.

Life becomes more direct, simple, real. We find ourselves becoming increasingly peaceful, healthy, happy, and harmonious, without any kind of big fuss. Our work is not yet over, but our minds are not so distracted by superficial worries. We lessen our petty attachments and selfish desires, enabling us to live in the world in a dutiful but carefree manner. The prince attains his birthright and comes to live in a palace of spiritual consciousness. Seated on a throne built of the gold of devotion, he presides over a kingdom of love. Thus is true royalty.

Problems

A man is driving down a road and his car develops a flat tire. He doesn't have a jack, so he is forced to walk to a nearby farmhouse to ask for help. All this causes him to become grouchy and curse his fate. Why should he have to suffer this inconvenience? Why should he have to walk all this distance for help? What if the farmer doesn't have a jack? What if the farmer has a jack but won't let him borrow it? What if the farmer sets his dog on him? What if, what if, what if . . . ?

By the time the guy makes it to the farmhouse, he has worked himself into a real snit. He's angry about everything and everyone. He's convinced that the world is out to get him. He knocks on the door, the farmer answers, and all our friend can blurt out is, "Keep your stupid jack; I don't need your help anyway!"

Baba Hari Dass has written, "The world is not a burden; we make it a burden by our desires. When the desires are removed, the world is as light as a feather on an elephant's back." What a vision. What a challenge.

How many of us feel that the world is as light as a feather? For many, life is a series of burdens and problems—health, family, career, politics, money, sex . . . Worse, no sooner do we resolve one difficulty than two or three more pop up. Feeling like soldiers walking across a minefield, we do our best to avoid conflicts but still find "it's always something." The world oppresses us, and it seems the best we can hope for is to compromise our dreams and settle for a life that, if we're lucky, is relatively safe and secure.

The issue of suffering is really one of responsibility because, as a result of our own desires and attachments, we create the chains that bind us like prisoners to objects, people, and situations. Our minds become petty, and we are happy only when we get what we want. Even then our happiness is short-lived. We feel victimized by a world in which we are powerless, a world which wends its way regardless of our wishes and what we may define as "good." A universe of unanswered questions, intrusive phenomena, and random pain carries us along in a chaotic swirl. Every sensitive person who is not planted firmly on the spiritual path will admit that, at one time or another, suicide may seem worth contemplation.

Into this dismal situation comes a message of light and hope from the great yoga masters: the world is not the cause of our burdens; the cause is in within our own minds. The suffering that we experience is not the result of the world's agenda to destroy us; it results from the manner in which we approach the world. By shifting our orientation, the world can appear as a beautiful place, filled with grace, sweet joys, and love. This is not to imply that life becomes a bowl of cherries. But when one perceives the spiritual reality underlying all events, life becomes meaningful, purposeful, and satisfying. Spiritual perception does not come by wearing rose-colored glasses over our eyes; it arises from removing the dirt-smeared goggles we currently see through.

In our society it is considered normal to be stressed-out and overwhelmed. It is a rare person who lives with good health and inner peace, who does not hold grievances against others, and who works at a satisfying job which contributes to society. We complain that we wish to be happy, but we refuse to undertake the spiritual work that can provide us with what we say we want. I've come to believe this is because spiritual teachers demand accountability, while we want commiseration. We abhor the message that our lives are of our own making. We yearn to hear that the world is a horrible place in which splendid people like ourselves are misunderstood and mistreated by those who do not belong to the proper social, political, or religious clique.

Like our friend with the flat tire, we create many hells for our-selves as a result of the unhealthy use of our minds. Our minds constantly chatter, broadcasting messages of hurry, worry, fear, and self-doubt. We've gotten stuck on the treadmill of attraction and repulsion, exhausting ourselves in a vain attempt to boost our damaged self-esteem. We've gotten into such a state that when we meet someone who tells us we are responsible for our own lives, we protest in knee-jerk fashion this isn't possible.

The spiritual teacher is like a generous farmer, happy to lend us his jack and show us how it works. He will not actually do the work for us, for that is our duty. How supported we feel, though, knowing that he has changed many flats and can appreciate and respect our situation. He points out possible problems that might arise and cautions us to be sure to tighten the lug nuts so that when the job is done we can continue on our journey. His goal, and ours, is not to have us spend the rest of our lives changing tires. He is simply there to help us get further down the road in a vehicle which runs on all cylinders and has its wheels firmly on the ground. And for this help, we smile in glad astonishment, all we needed to do was ask.

All of us, in one way or another, have flat tires in our lives. The choice about how to address our problems is ours to make. We can moan and groan about how unfair the world is, or we can choose to take responsibility for our situation, have the humility to ask for guidance, and then go about doing the work necessary to become free. Free will means we can choose between clinging to our ego-centered problems or walking the spiritual path of compassion, detachment, and service. I think God is a genius for creating a universe in which we are presented such a simple choice.

Ishtadeva

In yoga practice, an aspirant may worship a form of God as a means of making accessible the One formless Absolute. This chosen form of God is called one's *Ishtadeva*. The only means of determining one's Ishtadeva are through one's own heart and through experiences that may arise on the spiritual path. This is the story of my experience with my Ishtadeva.

In 1979, I had a profound experience in my apartment in Newark, Delaware, while listening to water boil in a teapot. Perhaps the rather mundane circumstances and the unexpected nature of the experience confirm that God truly is omnipresent and will communicate to us wherever we might be. Once in a while you *can* be shown the light in the strangest of places if you look at it right.

As I listened to the water begin to boil, I was presented with a vision of the entire human population—past, present, and future—in a type of pyramid of consciousness. At the bottom of the pyramid were the large majority of human beings: mundane personalities involved in mundane affairs. As the water in the teapot heated and produced sound, the energy seemed to spur my vision, and I ascended higher in the pyramid. I saw that as the pyramid rose and became more narrow, there were fewer human beings, but they were of a more magnanimous and spiritual character.

As the sound and energy of the teapot increased, I saw that different members of the human race had ascended to higher and higher levels of spiritual accomplishment. The higher realms included yogis and saints of all religions. As the water reached its boiling point and as it whistled through its lid, I saw the very top of the pyramid, the pinnacle of humanity. There I saw one person, Jesus.

For a long time I was reluctant to discuss this vision because the last thing I wanted was for people to think I was yet another dogmatist claiming that Jesus Christ is the greatest of all saints, the only son of God, whom you must accept to save you from your sins, blah, blah, blah. As I hope this essay will make clear, one's experience of his or her Ishtadeva is just that: a unique, personal experience that cannot be generalized and certainly should not be used as a weapon of intolerance and judgment.

For many years, I had difficulty acknowledging the reality of the presence of my Ishtadeva in my life. Besides my aforementioned reluctance to contribute to our society's Christian prejudice and misunderstanding, I was also, to be quite frank, turned off by the whole Jesus image. It was not until I got beyond the image to the reality itself that I became able to bask in the grace of this divine elder brother.

In sadhana, I had worked with different forms of the One formless God, and I had found growth and support in each of these. Yet each time I climbed towards the summit of devotion to one of these forms, I found Jesus at the end of the road. This is not to say that my journeys were wasted time. Hardly, for they each provided me with a series of experiences and a set of tools which clarified and solidified my spiritual identity and ability to teach and heal. In addition, the spiritual teachers I have studied under, though they may have had different Ishtadevas, are my beloved mentors who have made possible the degree of God-consciousness I now experience. They each showed me, in their own way, that a path is only as good as the student who walks it and that all paths lead to the Self. We find our true Self at the end of our chosen path by meeting, and then merging with, our personal Ishtadeva.

The concept of Ishtadeva, of a personally chosen form of God, may be difficult to grasp for many Westerners. We have been presented with a cultural myth which purports very dictatorially that there is only one true image of God—that of the stern but somehow loving Father. We have also been told that creating images of God is idolatrous, with some societally approved exceptions such as Christmas displays.

Such cultural myths are obviously chauvinistic and appear as such when seen in the light of many of the world's cultures, particularly that of India. In India, the devout feel free to worship any of literally thousands of images of Gods and Goddesses. They may or may not believe theoretically that there is One Supreme God in these various forms. Regardless, each individual is welcome to choose a form attractive to him or her. It is even said light-heartedly that there exists a different form of God for each Hindu.

This, again, may offend our Western sensibilities, especially when we are confronted with the characteristics of some of these Divine Beings. Many of them are kind, but others are wrathful. Some are ascetic, others quite lascivious; some care about human beings, others play with humanity as if we were made for their amusement. Others do not resemble the Divine in any way our Western minds could imagine: there are monkeys, fish, boars, and deities with several heads, arms, and legs. But monotheism simply means there is only one God; it does not mean that God will appear to all people in the same way.

If an ordinary American teenager can receive a revelation of Christ while listening to water boil, perhaps others can receive their experience of God by worshipping in a way that does not make sense to our Western conditioning. Here, perhaps, lies the lesson for us. For too long we of the Judeo-Christian culture have been operating under the assumption there is an absolute truth which is in our sole possession. Considering how many foolish mistakes we make in matters far less transcendent, I suggest we critically consider the notion that we alone have access to the one ultimate, final Truth.

For anyone of a devotional nature, establishing a relationship with one's Ishtadeva is a great boon to spiritual development. My experience with my Ishtadeva, Jesus, has taught me the demands and gifts of devotion. These include the willingness to acknowledge his presence, in spite of my desire to hide, and to accept his guidance, in spite of my desire to ignore it.

To meet your Ishtadeva it is necessary to release pre-conceived ideas and expectations about yourself and God. Dive into your heart, explore the ways that God speaks to you, and play with different manners in which you are comfortable relating to God. Use your imagination and allow it to grow into intuition. Then nurture your intuition until it blossoms into the realization that God is here to speak with you, walk with you, and guide your every step.

Forgiveness

In virtually all meditative traditions, one finds instructions to "release" thoughts, "let go" of attachments, and "cease clinging" to likes and dislikes. These verbs imply that a quiet mind is not so much something gained or accomplished but something already existing, underlying our present chaotic condition. The quiet mind is revealed when we loose ourselves from binding impediments, such as grievances against others.

I was at a yoga retreat a number of years ago, where a woman asked Baba Hari Dass a question about an interpersonal problem that had plagued her for some time. Babaji told her that the answer to her dilemma was to let go of the problem.

She sat quietly for a moment, and I could see that his words had deeply penetrated her mind. Suddenly her eyes lit up. As they say, she "got it!" In awe and wonder, she asked, "You mean . . . it's that simple?" "Yes," the guru responded with a chuckle.

As if unsure of her immense good fortune, she double-checked, "It's really that simple?" What could Babaji do but smile sweetly and reassure her, "Yes, it is that simple."

It may be that simple for a master yogi, but it certainly doesn't seem that simple, or at least that easy, for us. What is it that keeps us so trapped in emotional suffering, in dissatisfaction, in a guilt-ridden past and a fearful future? My observation is that we have an uncanny resistance to forgiving and forgetting, a drunken unwillingness to release the past and its hangover on our present.

We tend not to see other people in the present. We "hold them to a place," defining them based on previous experiences. We fail to permit them the grace to change, to grow. Instead, we anticipate that their personalities will remain static. Our beliefs then become a self-fulfilling prophecy. Even if others do change for the positive, we refuse to acknowledge their growth by clinging to their past. Thus our relationships remain stuck.

Forgiveness is generally thought of as some special grace that we bestow upon others. First, we interpret someone's behavior as damaging to us or those with whom we identify. Then, out of the supposed magnanimity of our hearts, we give them a break and bestow our forgiveness upon them. I think forgiveness is actually more of a relinquishing of our victim consciousness. Forgiveness is a willingness to release all of our reasons, no matter how seemingly righteous, that keep us from peace. Forgiveness helps us get our power back, reminding us that we are the source of our own experience of the world.

This doesn't mean that bad things don't happen to generally good people or that we have to meekly accept everything that is directed our way. Free will means we can deliberately choose the environments and beings with whom we would like to share our lives. Most of us have very little free will, however, because we are pushed and pulled by our attractions and repulsions, many of which are unconscious, into experiences over which we have little control. Through forgiveness, we come to recognize that our own consciousness is the origin of our experience. With this recognition, our personal power to control the flow of events in our lives increases, and we garner a certain potency over the manifestation of our world.

Spiritual practice produces the awareness that we are not our bodies. We are consciousness, within which thoughts arise and pass away, similar to the way clouds appear and disappear in the empty sky. As we realize our existence as separate from passing mental conditions, we garner a willingness to release negative thoughts. Security is not obtained by fighting negative thoughts but by realizing that our identity is not threatened by releasing them. The sky exists regardless of the presence of clouds.

We can learn to see that grievances and condemnation bring suffering and that forgiveness delivers peace. Then we can choose what brings us peace and release what causes us to suffer. One doesn't have to be a great genius to participate in this process. One does, however, need to be willing to let go of blame and guilt allied with the past and anxieties and fears associated with the future. The peace we are seeking cannot be found in yesterday or tomorrow. The past is a memory and the future mere imagination. Forgive your brothers and sisters, forgive yourself, forgive God, and "be here now," in the peace and spacious freedom that forgiveness provides.

The Great Trinity

A contemporary Zen master, John Daido Lori, has said that for an aspirant to progress on the spiritual path, he or she will need Great Faith, Great Doubt, and Great Determination. I capitalize these qualities in an effort to represent the magnitude of the spiritual undertaking. We are not referring to faith, doubt, or determination as they might influence a personal belief system. Rather, we are examining the attitude one must develop in order to undertake the process of transformation of consciousness.

Faith and doubt are like two fire sticks. Determination is the energy which rubs them together, producing a spark. Lacking any one of these three qualities, there will be no "fire," and the result will be a lopsided approach to spirituality.

Faith is based on a quality of trust. Ultimately it is a trust in oneself—in our ability to find a path, to practice diligently, and to achieve our goal. We project our trust onto our teachers, allowing them to reflect back to us what we are capable of attaining. Faith is not based on adopting correct belief systems; it does not mature through dogma or blind acceptance. Faith is developed by recognizing the next step in one's path of growth, and then taking what feels like a leap in that direction, letting go of all that seems certain and secure at our present stage. My experience is that this leap of faith is challenging and somewhat scary every time it is taken. By repetition of the process, however, one can recognize that it really is safe. In fact, instead of falling, faith leaves one free to fly.

Doubt, though condemned by the orthodox who need to cling to established belief structures, can actually be a tremendous asset to an aspirant. Healthy doubt reflects a degree of the confidence, independence, and self-respect that one needs to progress on the spiritual path. There is no use denying doubts in order to be "good."

Truth is not so fragile that it cannot endure in the face of our probing. It is dogmatism, not truth, that demands that someone passively absorb a teaching preached by another who claims to know more.

In the Old Testament, Jacob arrived at his transformation after a night spent wrestling with an angel. Likewise, we must honor our doubts and wrestle with them until they are resolved. Doubt is only a problem when it is allowed to degenerate into cynicism and inertia. Nothing is ever going to be perfect in our eyes, and no time is going to seem ideal. We should not use doubt as a justification for not doing our spiritual work.

Determination is the willingness to apply oneself in an energetic way to one's practice. The sticks of faith and doubt may be strong and sturdy, but without the application of some elbow grease we will continue to remain in the dark. Most of us don't have a problem with too much determination, though, but with too much laziness. We want someone else to do our work for us. The greatest teachings may be available to us, but it is we who must practice.

Baba Hari Dass has said that a teacher can cook, but only the student can eat for himself. It does not satisfy hunger to sit around and read a menu or to debate whether others have eaten or not. When you're hungry, you must eat your own meal. Those I have known who have progressed far on the spiritual path have been passionate in their practice. Sometimes one might even need to be overly daring to break through to the next stage of one's journey.

I do not believe that spiritual development is about wrapping ourselves in a cocoon of ease and support. It seems more like living in a blazing fire which burns away impurities. With Great Faith, Great Doubt, and Great Determination, it is possible to live in that fire and actually experience it as a nurturing, protecting, and guiding presence. Then our steps on the path will be steady and balanced, and we will come to know the security, freedom, and energy of spiritual life.

East and West

Someone said something interesting to me the other day. She said she wasn't interested in yoga because it is too "Eastern." Certainly she should be respected for her opinion and orientation. At the same time, however, it is obvious she doesn't understand the scientific nature of spirituality.

From a practical point of view, yoga, which means "union," may be understood as a verb. Yoga is a series of practices whereby one purifies his body, emotions, and thoughts in order to realize, or have union with, his true nature, the Self. While the yoga practices we are familiar with originated with the great sages of India several millennia ago, yoga is no more Eastern because it came from India than the law of relativity is Jewish because it was formulated by Albert Einstein.

Imagine you are learning to be an airplane mechanic. If the airline sends you to South America for training, your boss might tell you to report to work in a t-shirt and to bring along a thermos of cold lemonade. He might also tell you to be sure to check the cooling units on the plane, because they have a tendency to overheat. If you were learning the same trade in Siberia, you might be told to wear long johns to work and bring along some hot coffee. Your boss might warn you to be alert to the heating mechanisms in the plane, because the engine can get too cold to operate properly.

The principles and operation of getting the plane in the air safely have nothing to do with culture or personality. The differences in approach are rational, having to deal with practical considerations. The science of aerodynamics has nothing to do with whether the plane was built in South America or Russia.

We in America have a wonderful outlook whereby we believe

that anything wrong can be corrected. Hopefully this will lead us to resolve our political and social problems (or at least get the airlines to run on schedule). A difficulty arises, however, when we arrogantly assume that if we don't like something, our opinion is conclusive evidence that *it* needs to change. This approach is not going to work when we wish to learn a spiritual science.

Spirituality is as precise as mathematics. Our opinions, likes, and dislikes do not alter its laws. A great teacher said that spiritual discipline is the thing that people most avoid. But, he said, it is the ultimate refuge of everyone when they get tired of suffering. When we see that all our self-created plans, ideas, and concepts fail to bring us peace, then we turn to those teachings which are greater than ourselves.

It amazes me how much resistance we have in this country to learning spirituality from a teacher. In every other endeavor we seem to understand the need for a teacher or mentor, but when it comes to spirituality we seem to think it is a "do it yourself" job. While it is true, as Ramana Maharshi put it, "God, Guru, and Self are One," there are very few capable of this realization without instruction and guidance. If you think you have the intelligence, courage, inspiration, determination, and wisdom to succeed on the spiritual path without a teacher, well, you might consider your attitude is definite proof of your need! In addition, I think it a beautiful phenomenon that Nature has so arranged things that students need teachers. In this way, an extraordinarily sweet and powerful relationship can be formed: a relationship which can lead the student to appreciate God within and without.

Rather than forming biased opinions about things we don't understand and instead of seeking to change systems of practice which have proven their success over centuries, let us try to be humble and admit that we don't know everything. If we are not ready to submit to the self-introspection and discipline required of spirituality, so be it. Let us at least be honest enough to say that our interests lie elsewhere. But let us not fool ourselves into thinking that we are some special exemption to the rules which have guided great aspirants in every place and time throughout history.

Relationships

A man goes to a spiritual teacher and is told, "God is inside every living being." Thrilled with this new knowledge, the fellow walks home repeating to himself, "God is inside all beings, God is inside all beings, God is inside . . ." Suddenly startled from his reverie, he hears someone yelling, "Look out! A wild elephant is stampeding down the road. Move away or you'll be trampled!"

Forcing himself to remain still, he concentrates on God being inside of the elephant and refrains from running away. The elephant comes charging down the road, coming closer and closer to our stationary hero. Then, at the critical moment, the elephant doesn't pause at all, it tramples right over him.

The man, battered and beaten, returns to the spiritual teacher and complains, "You told me God was inside every being. I looked for God inside the elephant, so why was I trampled?" The teacher replied, "Looking for God in the elephant was good, but you failed to heed God in the form of the person who told you to run away."

Relationships don't work. That's the bad news or the good news, depending on how you look at it. Relationships don't work when they are given an assignment they can't fulfill: that of making us feel complete. The failure of relationships may appear as bad news because we experience pain when they end. The fact that relationships fail, however, is actually good news, because this highlights the futility in trying to attain happiness outside ourselves. The failure of relationships can serve as a fierce, but effective, reminder that the peace and positive energy we seek must be found within.

Many of us have had the experience of meeting someone and falling headlong into infatuation with their poise, radiance, and beauty. After a few dates, or perhaps a few years, we can hardly believe that our Prince Charming or Princess Bride turns out to be, actually, not much more than an imperfect human being. At that point we have a choice. We can accept responsibility for our erroneous perceptions and expectations, forgive the other for being more like ourselves than we care to admit, and get to work on clearing the garbage that prevents us from experiencing love. Or, we can imagine that the problem is due to the fallibility of the other person, and we can condemn that person until the cows come home in order to justify our righteous, negative opinion.

The world reflects back to us our attachments and selfish desires. A man buys a new car and is proud as punch. He washes it and protects it from scratches, dents, and dogs who might pee on the wheels. Then he sells the car to his neighbor. Now he doesn't care what happens to the car. Did anything change about the man or the car? No, only his idea of ownership and how this supported his sense of identity.

When this idea of ownership, and its accompanying ego support, arises in relationship to other living beings, problems inevitably follow. When we identify with a certain person or group with whom we feel a kinship, we end up excluding others. We establish a circle of compassion in our minds in which we agree to squeeze in so many and no more. This is why we can sleep at night while people are starving to death but we get upset when much less critical problems befall our family or friends.

When we form cliques, we limit our willingness to experience relationship and, therefore, to know love. For love is not love until it is complete, whole, and universal. In the heavenly choir, everyone's voice is essential, and each has a note to sing, without which there is no whole. To exclude anyone from the circle of heaven is to misperceive the nature of divine love, which is, in a very deep sense, all for one and one for all.

There's currently a lot of talk about community. People are longing for a sense of connection to their family and neighbors. Much of this is an intelligent search for a more practical way to live. Seeking community has a rub, though, because we're still stuck in a pattern of looking to others to provide the remedy for the dissatisfaction we feel exists within ourselves. Beginning with an inner sense of lack, we seek that which will make us complete. When we cannot find it in people or objects, we become frustrated.

This dissatisfaction, ultimately, cannot be solved by rearranging people or things in our lives because it has its roots in the spiritual realm. Our personal unhappiness is the manifestation of our inability to relate to the Divine within, and our social malaise is our collective inability to relate to the Divine in each other. Our feeling of separation from others is the reflection of a deeper feeling of separation from God.

The potential for right relationships arises when we get to the essence of community—communion. Communion is a blending of consciousness, a surrender of individual ego identities in a space of spiritual devotion. Communion comes when we are willing to purify our minds and hearts so that we no longer project our attachments and selfish desires onto others. This means taking responsibility for our anger, judgments, and grievances and releasing these negative emotions through forgiveness and compassion.

With communion, life grows from a constant struggle to get what we want and avoid what we detest to an increasingly graceful dance of relating to God in life's various situations. In a spirit of unity, we seek to perceive the one Divine Being who resides in all hearts. In a spirit of diversity, we seek to honor the dance of relationships by interacting and relating to others in a healthy and appropriate manner. We learn from spiritual teachers, run from wild elephants, and pray, dance, sing, and have as much fun as possible with the other members of our human family.

Namaste

One of the most striking aspects of yogic philosophy is the teaching that the mind is not, in itself, conscious. The mind is an insentient reflector of consciousness. Its activity reflects consciousness in somewhat the same fashion that the activity of a compass reflects the presence of magnetic impulses. In the West, we tend to believe Descartes' famous assertion: *cogito, ergo sum* (I think; therefore I am). To the yogi, thoughts actually cloud the essence of who "I" am. The quest for realization is an effort to go beyond thought, beyond conditioned mind, to experience the source of consciousness. Spirituality begins where thought ends.

According to yogic philosophy, consciousness is of the nature of a pure "I" sense. As this "I" associates with different forms of insentient nature, such as the body and mind, these forms appear to be independently conscious. In fact, the body does not walk, the breath does not breathe, the mind does not think without the presence of the activating consciousness.

There is a famous Zen question, "Is the taste of tea in the tea leaves or in the tongue?" In other words, does one's experience of the world arise as a result of external stimuli or from internal response? From a yogic perspective, the taste of tea is a collaboration between the tea and the tongue. As Claude Bragdon put it, our experience of the world is a collaborative effort of both receptivity and creativity.

The collaboration resulting in our experience of the world goes something like this. First, the senses receive stimuli from the external environment, conveying this information to the mind. The mind then translates this information into cognizable forms, and later adds personal biases to this neutral information.

Take the example of a person looking at a sunset. The eyes see a form of mass, light, and color. This pure stimuli received by the eyes is sent to the part of the mind called *manas*, which collates sensory information. Manas replicates, to the best of its ability, the impressions fed by the senses, reproducing an image of the external world—in this case, an image of the sunset. The intellect, or *buddhi*, then identifies the perception: "This is a sunset." The final pronouncement is made by the ego, called *ahamkara*, which is essentially judgmental, proclaiming the sunset good or bad, pleasurable or painful, acceptable or unacceptable (and other sets of the pairs of opposites) based solely on personal inclination.

The nature of one's reality is highly personal, vastly subjective. Everyone's mind and senses, just like fingerprints, are different. In addition, the external world is always in a state of flux. Every single perception is sole and unique, arising from the interchange between an individual's one-of-a-kind mind and senses (the perceiver) and a once-in-a-moment external world (the perceived).

No two living beings experience the world identically. In general terms, human minds experience a certain range of sensory data whose parameters are relative to other living creatures. We see fewer colors than bumblebees, for instance, and we have a smaller range of hearing than cats. In more specific terms, one's human ego apprehends the world relative to those of other human egos. What one person deems beautiful and interesting is to another person hideous and a waste of time. This is why there is such vast disagreement as to what is attractive, what is art, what is socially acceptable, and what is moral.

Some Eastern systems terminate with this analysis of perceiver and perceived and conclude that all is ephemeral and that there is no axis upon which changing perceptions revolve. Devotional schools of yoga go further; they say there exists an Absolute Reality which is eternally present as the underlying basis of all transient, individual experiences. There is an Absolute Consciousness, an Awareness, a Divine Center, from which the universe arises and by which it is sustained. It is this ocean into which the many rivers of individual experience flow. It is this Supreme Consciousness which we call God.

We honor God, transcendent and immanent, when we say "*namaste*." Namaste is a traditional Indian greeting which literally means "I honor you." On a more esoteric level, it also means that when you go deeply enough into your consciousness and I go deeply enough into mine, we find that we are One. This One appears as many in the realm of mind and senses, but on a deeper level all things are united in the One. This One is the source, sustainer, and eventual completion of all form. We can never leave our source because our source is always with us, as us.

Our problems arise because we feel ourselves separate from the One, from God. From the standpoint of the suffering human being, this separation feels tragic. From the standpoint of the One, the separation is illusory. How can the waves ever be separate from the ocean?

Through spiritual practice we can quiet the tumultuous distractions in our minds and deeply feel in our hearts the reality of the unity of consciousness. Then our separative suffering naturally evaporates, like clouds before the warmth of the sun. Life ceases to be an existential burden, and we awaken to discover ourselves interconnected with all living beings. Everywhere, in all forms and beyond form, is the One found expressing the purpose of divine love. Namaste.

Actions

Three men see a homeless little girl, and each is moved by her plight. The first recognizes the social and political influences that result in her fate. He sees the pain of the child but is so consumed with his own life and burdens that he cannot find a way to help. The second man perceives the same influences plus he understands the law of karma, of cause and effect, so he appreciates the predicament of the child from a vaster perspective. As a person of some wisdom, he expresses his compassion by donating a portion of his time and resources to easing her plight.

The third man understands the viewpoints of the other two, but he also sees the child as no different from his very self. He knows her pain because he knows his own pain. His desire to help arises spontaneously, without rational survey, just as his right hand would help his left hand should it fall into a fire. Whether he can practically assist or not, a tenderness born of recognized identity arises in his heart, and he longs to do all he can to eliminate her suffering.

The yogic tradition refers to three types of actions: *karma, dharma,* and *seva.* These are the three ways of responding to life, and they are based on the manner in which we perceive ourselves and the world. Karma and dharma are closely related, and in a sense they are actions which are required of us by nature, by social law, or by conscience. Seva is activity of a different quality, however, occurring as a result of spiritual maturity.

The term "karma" has entered colloquial usage and, like most subtle concepts that have become popularized, it is mostly misunderstood. Country and Western singer Willie Nelson had a hit song in which the chorus went, "It really ain't hard to understand/If you want to dance you got to pay the band/Just a little ol' fashioned karma goin' round." Willie's right about paying for the band, but that's not the whole story.

Karma literally means action and is used in yogic texts to designate the binding nature of action. Action is binding because of the law of cause and effect, which provides that every cause will eventually have an effect upon the causal agent. This means that all of our thoughts, words, and deeds will result in consequences suitable to our intention and energy extended. Most action is binding because it perpetuates the cycle of cause and effect, pleasure and pain, life and death.

On a microcosmic level, each individual generates his own karma as a result of selfish drives that arise from the conscious or subconscious areas of the mind. On a macrocosmic level, karma is Nature's means of balancing the books, ensuring that like provides for like. Karma ensures that there are no errors, that nothing is gained that is not deserved, and that until spiritual growth makes the will powerful enough, very little takes place in our lives outside the parameters of cause and effect.*

Dharma is a fascinating concept with a multitude of connotations. In the field of ethics, dharma signifies virtue and righteousness; dharma is the doing of what is right and the avoidance of what is wrong. Although there are a few general principles of dharma in yoga—such as non-violence and truthfulness—it is understood that each individual has his own dharma unique to his life situation.

Dharma is the acceptance of obligation and the undertaking of duty, both personal and social. Dharma is the fulfillment of the law of karma, recognizing the need for right action, right speech, and right thought if individuals and societies are to be healthy and prosperous. To follow one's dharma is to hear the beat of one's own drummer, knowing that this inner rhythm is in harmony with the cosmic drum in every heart. To act in a dharmic manner is the antithesis of the selfish egoism which insists on the fulfillment of pain-producing desires. To be dharmic is to be sensitive enough to intuit what is right and to have the courage to walk that path.

A dharmic person is good-hearted, but it takes more than this to break the shackles of cause and effect. For being good, though an improvement on being selfish, is still limiting, since good acts also have their effects. What we might call good karma is every bit as binding as what we call bad karma. Gold chains bind the prisoner as tightly as those made of iron. To shatter all chains, seva is needed.*

Seva simply means service, traditionally to one's teacher or community, but it also carries a deeper connotation. It is service above and beyond the call of necessity (karma) or duty (dharma). It is service offered out of love. Seva is the offering of one's self into service of the Self that we all share. As such, it is an affirmation of unity. Seva places what is part in service to the whole. Seva is the fuel that keeps the fire of love alive.

Seva is the offering of oneself as a natural response to suffering in the world in the same way that the sunflower naturally lifts its head to the sun. It is service without intent for reward, recognition, or even personal betterment. It arises from love for God within one's own heart, and it is offered to the God of love that lives in all hearts.

Seva transcends the cycle of cause and effect because it is transpersonal action, undertaken without personal motivation or concern. Seva arises spontaneously, and one feels as if acts are being accomplished through him rather than by him. It's sort of like being Jerry Garcia's guitar; it was an important part of the show but certainly doesn't deserve any of the applause. The divine maestro is the one playing through the instruments of our bodies and minds, performing the great acts of seva. Karma makes life a scripted journey, dharma makes life a battle for right, while seva makes life a dance.

We all find ourselves confronted with internal and external problems. How we view ourselves will determine how we see those trials and will precipitate how we respond. To live only within the boundaries of karma is prison. To live only within the boundaries of dharma is society. To live for seva, though, is to live a life without boundaries—in other words, to be free. Let us be honest with ourselves and acknowledge where we are at in the various spheres of our lives, and then let us continue our work and prayer that we may transform our every action into an act of seva.

*See the essay entitled "Karma" for a more complete analysis of this phenomenon.

Beliefs

A learned professor wished to cross the river, so he engaged the services of a common ferryman. As the ferryman rowed his small craft, the professor asked his opinion on the government's economic policy. The ferryman apologized to the professor, explaining that he was an uneducated man who had never learned the principals of economics. "A pity," exclaimed the professor, "for without a knowledge of economics one cannot succeed in the field of investment. My dear man, you have wasted a quarter of your life."

To continue the conversation, the professor asked the ferryman what he thought of the latest styles of clothing that people were wearing. The ferryman again apologized, as he was forced to explain that he was a poor man who did not have the resources needed to keep abreast of fashion. "A shame," pronounced the professor, "for without a knowledge of how to dress appropriately, one cannot succeed in obtaining a high social position. My unfortunate friend, you have wasted half your life."

The professor then asked the ferryman his opinion of the country's ruling political party. The ferryman could only offer that he tried to stay updated on politics but he was a simple man who was mostly occupied with the affairs of his own family and community. "A disgrace," the professor exhorted, "for without a knowledge of political power one cannot succeed in attaining advantage over one's enemies. You poor soul, it seems you have wasted three quarters of your life."

Suddenly, a strong tide overturned the boat, and the two men were tossed into the water. "Swim for the shore!" yelled the ferryman. "I can't," cried the professor, "I don't know how to swim." "A true pity," thought the ferryman as he watched his passenger taken under by the current. "He lived by water but never learned to swim. He wasted his entire life."

Believing in God is a foolish thing. Disbelieving in God is also a foolish thing. The foolishness is not with God, however; it is inherent in the nature of belief. For beliefs are of the mind and, like all phenomena of the mind, are transitory, evanescent, and undependable.

Believing in God can be like believing in Santa Claus. One may find happiness, psychological comfort, and even companionship with others who share the same belief, but one day the belief is bound to pass away. Sooner or later the illusory image will be shattered. So, let us not depend on belief that has not been substantiated by concrete experience.

Disbelieving in God, on the other hand, seems to me to be only possible by denying the overwhelming evidence that a conscious principle underlies the entire universe. Not believing in God is akin to not believing in the sun. It may be possible to remain indoors all the time and therefore not experience the sun, but reality is not affected by one's hibernation.

Rather than believing or disbelieving, let us be honest and admit to not knowing. Rather than clinging to belief or disbelief as if they will keep us afloat on the tides of life's uncertainties, let us acknowledge how truly limited are our knowledge and experience. Certainty does not involve belief. If I ask you if you have fingers on your hands, you can answer with no doubt. No matter how many people say differently, regardless of political referenda, learned opinions, even holy scriptures, you know for yourself if you have fingers on your hands. It is simply not a matter of belief or disbelief.

So it should be in regard to our experience of God. The yogi passes beyond belief, hope, and imagination in an effort to communicate directly with the Supreme Consciousness. He does so as a result of a factual, repeatable process of purification and attunement. When Swami Vivekananda met Paramahamsa Ramakrishna, he asked him, "Have you seen God?" The master replied that he saw God more clearly than he saw the young man who was standing before him asking the question. This reality, devoid of fantasy, is religion; and yoga, devoid of superstition, is the science of religion.

Yoga offers a time-tested path for the direct realization of God, Goddess, Self, Truth—whatever name we superimpose on the Divine. Thousands of men and women have applied themselves to authentic processes of spiritual development and have succeeded in their quest. Mystical experience is, in a sense, the most down-to-earth phenomenon, because it is available to everyone as a birthright. What is mystifying is why so many people linger in unhappiness when peace and joy, or at least the path to peace and joy, beckons before us.

Life is short and distractions are many. We involve ourselves in activities which create confusion, stress, and despair. We spiral downward into depression, looking for a helping hand to lift our spirits high. And we seem to welcome almost any hand except one which points us back to ourselves and says, "It is your responsibility to lift yourself."

Our friend the professor had become so sidetracked by his various interests and accomplishments that he failed to learn what every person living near water should know. While our feet are planted firmly on the earth, it would seem wise for us to learn what every person who lives near the waters of death should know: Who am I? What is the purpose of my life? What will happen to me when I die?

To cling to immature religious beliefs not rooted in experience will not suffice. To believe that I can swim will not help me if I have not actually entered the water and learned what to do. Similarly, the cynic who claims that there is no spiritual reality because he does not know of it, is like saying that because he has never been swimming, neither has anyone else.

Yoga is a path to direct, personal experience of the Divine Consciousness, and anyone can taste of this reality if they are willing to apply themselves. If the professor knew he would one day fall into the water, it's a good bet he would have taken the time to learn how to swim. You and I are sure one day to fall before death. At that time the only knowledge that will be of value will be the wisdom gained by spiritual insight. Let us be candid and admit how little we know, and let us humbly apply ourselves to growing spiritually in order that we not waste our lives.

Why Do Bad Things
Happen to Good People?

Why do bad things happen to good people? To put it simply—they don't. The reason for this is twofold. First, who is a good person and who is a bad person? In reality, each of us is such a mixed bag of personality traits and ego quirks that it is impossible to place our entire persona in a box and label it as "good" or "bad." There's enough good in the worst of us and enough bad in the best of us to make it advisable to drop the judging, labeling, and finger-pointing and to offer compassion toward all.

Second, our determinations of what are "good" or "bad" events and circumstances frequently just reflect our limited and self-serving viewpoints. We call "good" that which satisfies our desires and "bad" that which thwarts our personal designs. To complicate matters further, our desires, and therefore the value systems with which we define good and bad, change over time. We have all had our satisfaction turn to lament shortly after getting what we were sure we wanted. Likewise, we have all had the experience of being deeply disappointed about a situation only to later appreciate the good fortune that arose out of what we first saw as misfortune.

In the West, it is difficult to find the broad, non-dogmatic spiritual outlook necessary to understand the relative and subjective nature of what we call good and bad. That is why most of us lack any realistic spiritual context within which we can honestly understand the events of our lives. The Abrahamic religions postulate a powerful deity who rewards good behavior and punishes bad behavior, in this life or in the great beyond. But among and even within these religions there is no consensus on what constitutes good and bad behavior. In addition, history shows that religious standards change over time. If yesterday's acceptable behavior were not today's sin, a Christian could still return home from church to a lunch prepared by a human slave.

The yogic tradition is less concerned with social relativities, focusing instead on a universal ethic. Ethics in yoga is a practical framework of attitudes and behaviors which brings human beings into harmony with the entire universe, rather than a set of dictates handed down by a theological authority. This is why the yogic tradition considers nature such a grand teacher: she is uncompromisingly harmonious. When we live in accordance with nature's rules, we prosper on every level. And what are these rules? Eat healthy food, exercise frequently, don't sweat the small stuff, and love your neighbor as yourself. These are not complicated dictates but guidelines based on common sense that everyone, in his or her heart, already knows to be true.

In the search for peace, one comes to value all experience, good or bad, pleasant or unpleasant—call it what you will—as potential for growth. Although it might be hard to grasp while undergoing a painful experience, isn't it true that growth often arises from difficulties? Since this is the case, perhaps we can become more enthusiastic about our troubles and see that they are the soil from which the bounty of life arises. It isn't so much a question of figuring out if something is good or bad; it's a matter of accepting our lives as they are and doing our best to respond with compassion, wisdom, and a sense of humor. It's not so much a question of judging who is a good or bad person; it's more a matter of recognizing the common spirit that runs through all of us.

Author and humanitarian Bo Lozoff has said that the reason most people are unhappy is that they live life in a superficial way, whereas life, by its very nature, is a deep and powerful mystery. Yoga practice is an art and science designed to bring about direct experience of the spiritual mystery of life. This often requires that we give up our habit of seeking easy, packaged answers. To advance in yoga practice and to find real satisfaction in life, it is necessary to be somewhat of a maverick. We must learn to use our intuition and discover our own answers based on personal experience. It is only direct experience that will give us the confidence and freedom to delve deeply into the mystery and find out what lies in life's depths.

We would do well to stop ruminating on dichotomies of good and bad and to plunge into life with all its complexities and mind-boggling paradoxes. Christ talked about a "peace which surpasses understanding." Go beyond trying to understand life—it is not something to be understood. Life is something to be lived!

Helen Keller said, "Life is either a great adventure or it is nothing at all." Great adventures are bound to include challenges, successes and failures, magnificent victories and giant blunders. When you let go of the need to define events as good or bad, you discover the profundity of all experience. When you release yourself and others from judgment and condemnation based on good and bad, you discover a spontaneity and security that seems miraculous.

Yoga is a path to a level of consciousness that lies beyond the flatland of hurry, worry, fear, and self-doubt. But getting here takes a leap of faith. So take a giant dive off the edge of the cliff of your personal security. The first few tries you might tumble to the ground. But, if you keep trying, you'll learn how to spread your own wings. You'll fly on the winds of spiritual consciousness. You'll tire of running on the treadmill of likes and dislikes, good and bad, judgments and moods. You'll enjoy spending more time in yoga consciousness, satisfied with the two great gifts of yoga, shanti and shakti. You won't be so concerned with analyzing which threads of experience are good and which are bad, because you'll have the vision to see the entire tapestry of life in all its profundity, mystery, and grandeur.

Bringing the Real into the Unreal

From the unreal, lead us to the real.
From darkness, lead us to light.
From death, lead us to immortality.

Above is an ancient prayer from the yogic tradition that is fascinating to me for several reasons. First, it states that our current level of consciousness is unreal, dark, and morbid. Second, it suggests there is a state that is real, light, and immortal. Third, the prayer is in the third-person plural, implying that the path from our current state to the latter state is undertaken communally. Let's examine these three aspects of this prayer and determine whether it has relevance for our lives and times.

To begin with, we are presented with the notion that our current state is unreal, illusory, not based in sanity. This is a difficult teaching at first as we all hold a certain resoluteness that we understand the hard facts of life and the way the world operates. Yogic philosophy presents a different vision of life and the world from that held by most people. Yoga says reality has three components: *satyam*, it is eternal; *shivam*, it is inherently kind; and *sundaram*, it is beautiful. Most of us do not actually experience ourselves, others, or our world as being eternal, kind, and beautiful. We are, therefore, living in an unreal state. This unreal state is a sort of mental illness known as *avidya* (spiritual confusion).

Since the illness of spiritual confusion is mentally based, the healing of the illness also takes place in the mind. The first step in this healing is to loosen our stubborn grip on the way we define people and events. We usually expend tremendous energy reinforcing a particular viewpoint about who we are and who others are in relationship to us. Instead, we must learn to recognize that this perception of the world is limited, relative, subject to change, and frequently not conducive to peace or joy. We also find our perception about the nature of reality often conflicts with someone else's perception. This difference in confused perspectives is, in essence, the birthplace of human conflict, from the ordinary little hassle to the immense conflict of war.

When I was growing up I was warned by adults around me that someday I was going to have to make my way in "the real world." This chastisement was intended to prepare me for life in a competitive and vicious world. As one of my relatives put it, only half-kidding, "Do unto others before others can do unto you." What we find in yoga is that this view of life as a battlefield is simply a misperception generated by minds in spiritual confusion. If we can remind ourselves that our anger, jealousy, and anxiety are formed on unreal, fear-based viewpoints, we have a better chance of walking the path that will lead us to the real vision of eternal kindness and beauty.

The darkness referred to in the second line of the prayer is indicative of the feeling of being small and alone in a big, uncaring world. Every one of us has had to deal with feelings of loneliness and impotency. In fact, the more mature and sensitive a person, the more painful is the loneliness. This loneliness, however, is a pathway to spiritual communion. It is a pathway to be honored, not avoided.

Too often we run from our loneliness, distracting ourselves with the latest and the greatest. The yogis encourage us to dive into the loneliness, face it with our full being, and find how the loneliness is born and develops. Then we see that it is based on bodily identification. By identifying ourselves solely with our physical bodies we are overlooking the vastness of our connection with everything in creation. It is as if a wave on the sea looked around and thought itself distinct and independent of all the other waves, vulnerable to the bigger waves and fearful of the calamity of being consumed by the ocean.

This brings us to the third line of the prayer, the transition from a consciousness of death to one of immortality. The key to transcending the sense of being just a wave and to feeling one's connection to the entire ocean is to de-program consciousness from physical identification. Virtually all of us identify ourselves almost exclusively with our bodies, with the result that our life story begins at a certain date and could end at any time, even without our consent. This identification with the body breeds a fear of death and, eventually, even a fear of change. We desire to live, to live well (as we define "well"), and to live securely. Life, however, is filled with change, and our desire for security brings us into opposition with very the nature of life.

To resolve this dilemma and transcend physical consciousness is not an easy matter. It takes a combination of practice and service. Practice means engaging in a consciousness-elevating technique, such as yoga generally or meditation in particular, on a regular, steady basis. This will help shift our awareness so that we become increasingly in touch with the vastness of our own being. We acknowledge that we have physical bodies, of course, while we also come into contact with our minds, hearts, and souls. Regular practice asks us to become disciplined, little by little, until practice becomes as regular and as ordinary as brushing our teeth.

Service is expressed in a willingness to steer our lives into an attitude of caring about others. One of my teachers taught that spirituality simply means giving more than you take. Becoming more of a giver and less of a taker is something accessible to all of us. Service helps us recognize that from one point of view we may be individual waves, but it is equally true that we are as one in the depths and that we rise and fall together.

This brings us to my third point of interest, the plural nature of this prayer. In the yogic tradition, *satsang*, gathering together for truth, is deemed an invaluable and necessary component of spiritual development. Invaluable because it is so precious to be with a group of people who are earnestly attempting to grow out of their selfishness and are willing to support one another; necessary because no one is intelligent and brave enough to progress on the spiritual path without assistance. It is a beautiful fact of nature that to grow out of our selfishness we need friends to help us and whom we can help in return.

In all too many social communities, people support each other's anger and grievances. Common enemies are identified and cliques are formed. In satsang, community is based on supporting each other in *sadhana* (spiritual practice) and *seva* (service to others). Spiritual practice is something we can all do. It doesn't have to be a big deal. Take ten minutes a day and dedicate it to cultivating wisdom and compassion.

The techniques you use may change with time while the development of wisdom and compassion will only deepen. If you take ten minutes a day for sadhana, at the end of the year you will have devoted sixty-two hours to your spiritual growth. You can't help but improve your quality of life with that kind of effort. And just imagine what our world would be like if more people spent sixty-two hours a year cultivating peace.

Seva, or service, is nothing less than learning how to feel good. If you believe you need to get in order to be happy, you will frequently find yourself miserable since there is always so much more to get. If you believe your happiness lies in giving, you will frequently find yourself joyful as there is always more to give. You don't need to be phony-holy or anything like that, just a little more considerate and kind. Don't underestimate the profound healing power of kindness. Expressing this innate kindness through service is a gift to others and to yourself.

For some twenty-five years I have been contemplating the opening prayer. At first it was just a seed of ideas, then it was a thorn that made me work and grow, and finally it has become a flower, constantly unfolding and revealing new beauty. For many of us this is an accurate description of yoga practice: learning a new skill, followed by regular practice, followed by ease and beauty.

Yoga is a path to the real, the light, and the immortal in you. Contemplate yogic ideas, develop a regular practice, and enjoy who you are. See you in class. Bring your reality!

The Guru

His job is to shed light, and not to master.
—Robert Hunter—

The invitation has arrived and you are thrilled to be invited to the big party. When the happy day arrives you dress in your finest attire and hop into your car. On the way to the gala event you realize, however, you don't quite know how to get to your destination. So you stop a friendly looking guy and ask for directions. He tells you that it's really fairly simple, though not necessarily easy, but if you follow his instructions you are certain to end up where you want to go.

Here, however, is where you start to act kooky. Instead of following his directions, you get out of your car and throw yourself at his feet, praising him as "The One Who Knows the Directions." The next day you come back with flowers and gifts, performing a ceremony in front of his house, intoning all that is holy in praise of "The One Who Knows the Directions." You return again and again, bringing your friends, preaching to your neighbors, telling them all about "The One Who Knows the Directions." The whole time you are making a big deal over the wrong thing, your songs of praise so loud you can't hear the gentleman softly asking, "Have you actually followed my directions and gone to the party?"

I can hardly think of anything more misunderstood on the spiritual path than the relationship of *guru* (teacher) and *chela* (student). The duty of the guru is to point in the right direction, and the duty of the chela is to walk in that direction. My experience is that there are many qualified teachers who properly point, but there are few students who actually walk.

There are two extreme states in the relationship of the student to his teacher. These are the classic imbalances in yoga known as "too little" and "too much." In "too little" consciousness, the individual makes a foolish assumption that he is intelligent and intuitive enough to travel the spiritual path on his own. The one who feels this way is making an arrogant evaluation about his own brains and brawn, one which will cost him time and energy in the long run. In addition, his conceit will ensure he does not receive an invitation to the big party (to continue our story) because everyone at the party has imbibed the great virtue of humility. To such a one who chooses to be his own teacher, the yoga tradition offers this counsel: "The one who is his own guru has a fool for a disciple."

In the "too much" mind, the individual engages in a hero-worship relationship with his teacher. Placing his teacher on a pedestal of unattainable accomplishment, he conveniently arranges an excuse not to perform the personal growth work required by the teacher. In addition, there is a subtle passive-aggressive dynamic at work whenever someone is placed on a pedestal. Those who place him there also secretly, subconsciously, want to knock him down. I have also seen here in the West that many aspirants have a unhealthy, imaginary "perfect parent" relationship with their guru. It's much easier, after all, to idolize a fantasy perfect mother or father figure than it is to do the work of healing the wounds that might exist in relationship to one's all-too-human and imperfect parents.

The guru is, truly, the greatest of human beings and deserves our love and respect. In our Western culture we honor those with good looks, lots of money, athletic skills, and political power. But the spiritually accomplished man or woman is the real success, the real hero. He is one who has attained the goal of creation. He has arrived at the summit of human attainment. He can serve as our role model and inspiration. His attainment, though, does not somehow magically transfer to us. We must proceed just as he did, performing spiritual disciplines and learning how to serve others.

Because the guru deserves our respect, we should treat him with a certain degree of deference. But, when you look in the guru's eyes, you can see a beautiful sparkle that says "love is only intimate between lovers." There is a balance, a yoga, to be found in our relationship to our teachers. We respect them as our spiritual elders, but we also let them lead us into the more intimate chambers of love between equals.

The fact that the guru is a living, breathing human being is also an important point. It is essential at some time in one's spiritual development to study with a living teacher. This enables one to receive personal instruction. Also a living teacher can help one's growth in a way that is almost unimaginable. A guru can push psychological buttons that the student doesn't even know he has. Someone once said, "A dead guru can't kick your butt." Plus, we can see that the teacher also lives in the world—he eats, sleeps, sweats, farts, and has to contend with Vermont's mosquitos. A historical guru or saint may be inspirational, but he is not of the same practical value to our lives. Babe Ruth can no longer help the Yankees win the pennant, and Jesus the carpenter can no longer repair your roof.

Finally, it's not essential that the guru be fully enlightened. First off, how would you know if he was? You'd have to be fully enlightened yourself to be able to recognize it in another. Secondly, few of us are spiritually mature enough to actually need an enlightened master. Most of us just need someone a little farther along the path, someone who is accessible, someone enough like us that he or she can understand our problems and help us take the next step on our journey. Besides, it doesn't matter how wise and loving is the guru. The honest question is: how wise and loving is the student?

A true guru doesn't want to make disciples, he wants to make enlightened, autonomous human beings. He only wants his students to enjoy the spiritual reality that he enjoys, the same one that was freely and joyously passed to him by his teacher. He doesn't want others worshipping him. How does this help anyone? The guru simply provides the directions and serves as living proof that the party is really taking place.

Martha and The Vandelles sang, "It doesn't matter what you wear, just as long as you are there." It doesn't matter what you wear to God's party. It doesn't matter what kind of vehicle you drive to get there. It doesn't matter who gave you directions. Techniques, religions, traditions—these are all fingers pointing the way. Let go of the attachment to staring at the finger; travel in the direction the finger is pointing. Use your guru's instructions to help you quiet your mind, open your heart, and learn how to serve others. This will take you where you want to go, to the great cosmic *lila* (party).

My personal experience is that the guru is the dependable friend who gives me the pat on the back or kick in the pants, whatever I need at the time. He doesn't want my thanks, my praises, my hallelujahs; he wants me to go to the party and have a great time. So if I want to express my gratitude to him, the only thing I can do is to become more like him, enjoying the party and lovingly serving others. Party on, Guruji!

Relax

Wake now!
Discover that you are the song that the morning brings.
—Robert Hunter—

The ashram was having a problem with mice, so the guru brought home a good cat. The cat did a fine job on the mice, but she became attached to the guru and followed him everywhere, even when he was performing his morning meditations. In order to keep the cat from disrupting his meditations, the guru took to tying the cat to a post.

The guru eventually died, and his students decided to continue with his "tradition" of tying the cat. The cat too later died, and a new cat was obtained so that she could now be tied to the post. The post rotted, so a new post was constructed in order that the cat could continue to be tied. Over successive generations different sects formed based on the type of cat to be tied, the type of rope to be used when tying, and the color paint used on the post. As you can imagine, today these sects are convinced they are following the founder's true teachings, while the other sects are ignorant blasphemers. Meanwhile, because the cats are always being tied, the mice enjoy the run of the ashrams.

One famous teacher confessed to "selling water by the banks of the river." How honest. Because all a real spiritual teacher does is reflect back to the student his inner being and the folly of his external search. Like the fabled musk deer that runs all over the forest searching for the beautiful fragrance, most students seem determined to run to exhaustion before collapsing on the ground and realizing the true source of the magnificent scent. All an authentic teacher can do is encourage the student in his pursuit and try to remind him that his own Self is what he is seeking.

The yogic tradition holds that every human being has a fullness within that is the source of love, joy, and peace. Called by different names, this source is one's true spiritual self, unscathed by the tribulations and hassles of life. Most people find it incredulous that their deepest identity is loving and peaceful, as we are more apt to experience ourselves as angry and stressed. The yogis acknowledge our present suffering but state that it is simply a superficial experience that arises due to a series of five psychological dynamics which are called *kleshas* (obstructions).

The first klesha is *avidya*, which refers to a primal ignorance. We'll return to the nature of this ignorance later, for now simply consider it the dynamic by which the individual forgets his intrinsic fullness. By the force of avidya, a feeling of emptiness arises as one forgets his spiritual identity. As a response to the pain of this forgetfulness, the second klesha, *asmita*, then occurs. Asmita is the creation of, and attachment to, a limited identity based primarily on biological and social conditioning.

Under the influence of asmita, an individual identifies himself with a set of definitions which narrow his ability to understand himself and relate to others. This is generally what we would call "ego," the feeling of being an isolated individual in an enormous world filled with those different from oneself. We see this in the way people feel estranged from those of "other" races, religions, or creeds. Asmita also generates a dualism which produces the third and fourth kleshas—*raga* (attraction) and *dvesha* (repulsion). Under raga and dvesha, we seek for those external objects and relationships which we incorrectly believe can fill the inner void, and we attempt to repel experiences and people who we believe can disrupt our lives. The end result of this process is the fifth klesha—*abhinivesha* (fear of change, especially the fear of death). This fear permeates our lives as we are afraid to let go of whatever security we feel we have. Abhinivesha produces an anxiety that things can always get worse, so cling tight to whatever little, tentative happiness you may chance to find.

Why do the kleshas exist? Why this wheel of life, with its incessant spin of life and death? Sensitive people often ask, "If God is all-powerful, couldn't He have created something more pleasant?" Why evil? Why pain? Why sickness? From the yogic perspective these are excellent questions. In fact, when these types of questions arise it is a sign the individual is developing a spiritual maturity. The next step is dealing with the answers.

I once had an argument with Baba Hari Dass, my yoga guru, about the nature of suffering. In front of a fairly large group of people, I put forth my premise that, basically, God is cruel. After all, if the best the creator can do is produce a world in which suffering and disappointment is the norm, in which cruelty can conquer kindness, and in which too many people feel life is passing by without answers to their deepest questions, well, maybe God is a jerk.

Hari Dass tried philosophy, he tried encouragement, he tried to ignore me, but I wouldn't let up. I wanted to know why suffering exists and how I could bring an end to it in my life! Finally, he said, "Relax; try to enjoy." At the time I was not satisfied with his answer. I closed my case with the pronouncement, "I will never worship whatever God created this world." I got up and left. Most of the audience was aghast at my seeming blasphemy and rudeness. Hari Dass chuckled, and even then I sensed that though he may not have been able to praise my understanding, he appreciated the passion of his student.

In the years since this event, I have learned that Hari Dass had given me a very profound teaching. Of course, it was one which, at the time, I did not have "the ears to hear." Fortunately, I have since realized that suffering and tension are two parts of the same coin.

They are like the wave and trough; they arise together in a code-pendent manner. The more we suffer, the more we grow tense. The more tension, the more we armor ourselves against the world and generate a self-fulfilling prophecy of increased suffering. It took years of practice before I could appreciate the wisdom of relaxing.

The world appears to us as an abode of suffering when we are under the influence of avidya, the primal ignorance. This igno-rance, however, is nothing more than a knot of tension deep in our being. Avidya is a phenomenon of nature that arises with creation. We may not appreciate all aspects of nature, but ours is not to evaluate but to learn how to live in harmony. Our task is not to de-stroy our ignorance, but to let it find its place in the totality of who we are. In this way we are kept humble. Because we acknowledge we are prone to mistakes, we can accept that we require guidance and supportive friends.

All of us, in the unenlightened state, are conditioned by the five kleshas. The suffering we experience under their influence is painful, but it also brings about a positive outcome. Suffering is nature's way of motivating us to seek for answers regarding the cause of suffering and its remedy. In the midst of tough times we certainly wonder if nature couldn't have perhaps come up with a better plan! But nature's plan is the divine plan, and through spiri-tual practice we can come to glimpse this plan and participate in its expression.

When we are tense we suffer. To relieve this suffering we chase after externals. This perpetuates the cycle of tension and suffer-ing. The way out is to undo the knots of tension. This is entirely an inner process. It will not be found in objects, in relationships, in churches, ashrams, or temples. It will not be found in tying up cats or buying water along the riverside. It will be found within you, as you. You are the song you are yearning to hear. Relax, hear its sweet song, try to enjoy.

Rest in Peace

The guru was giving a discourse before a group of attentive students. Suddenly, the assembly was interrupted by a woman rushing to the feet of the sage. Holding her lifeless child, she announced between sobs that her only baby was now dead. She declared her faith in God and the great sages and implored the guru to use his divine powers to restore the breath to her child. Filled with compassion but understanding the nature of life and the spiritual journey, the guru said he would perform the miracle if she could bring to him a mustard seed from a home that had not known suffering.

The woman raced frantically from house to house, imploring at each door the mustard seed that had not been within walls of suffering. But at each home the story was similar—poverty, illness, trauma, untimely death, always some calamity had made its way into the family. You can imagine how the despair of the grieving mother grew.

Exhausted and defeated, the woman eventually buried her child and returned to the guru. With a newfound understanding and humility she sat before the teacher, prepared to learn the lessons of life and death and the means to overcome suffering.

We in the West tend to believe in a myth that death will alleviate suffering. We fantasize that somehow the loss of the physical body results in consciousness being transported to a realm of rest and peace. Yoga does not agree that death ends suffering. Yoga believes strongly in reincarnation and the concept that the level of consciousness with which we leave this world will follow us to our next home. Yoga agrees that the post-life experience may be pleasant but says that it is not the permanent solution. Many people may have earned a stay in one of the heavenly realms, just as a hard-working laborer may earn two weeks vacation during the year, but both return to "work" at the conclusion of their respite.

The dead do not rest in peace any more than a vacationer is guaranteed his flights will arrive and depart on time. Death does not guarantee peace or wisdom. If someone leaves this world an angry, judgmental individual, there is no reason to believe he will suddenly awaken as an angel in a heavenly realm. Likewise, just because someone is temporarily living in a high sphere is no reason to believe that they are immensely wiser than we human beings. This is why yoga pays no heed to channeling, mediums, and other such phenomena.

Peace is not something that belongs to the dead; it is the goal of life. Resting does not mean lying beneath the ground; it means walking with your heart content. To rest in peace is not the result of death; it is the reward of a life well lived. Living well means strengthening the body, quieting the mind, opening the heart, and serving others.

The purpose of yoga practice is to learn to overcome suffering. For most of us, the first step in this journey is to alleviate bodily pains and discomforts. And this is no small step. It is very hard to care for much else when the body feels like a burden and one's vitality is lagging. However, after the body begins to stabilize, one sees how suffering is ultimately a spiritual problem that requires a spiritual solution. It is at this point that yoga begins to fulfills its potential as a spiritual therapy.

Many people in the West seek psychotherapy to help them cope with their problems and anxieties. Psychotherapy involves healing the *psyche*, the Greek word for soul. So psychotherapy should serve to heal the problems of the soul. The most common contemporary manifestations of the soul problem are hurry, worry, fear, and self-doubt.To deal with these four troubles, however, is to deal with symptoms and not the cause. The cause lays deep in the psyche as a primal idea which we in the West call sin.

In the West we have generally been taught that sin is a behavior that has somehow insulted the Supreme Being and for which we must pay a price, usually in the form of punishment. Yoga teaches that sin is simply the sense of separation from the one Creator and the unity of all life. But the individual soul can no more be separate from her creator than the wave can be separate from the ocean. As the wave is the expression of the ocean, the soul is the expression of the love of God. To believe and act from separation is not a sin, says yoga; it is just an illusion. And illusions require healing, not punishment.

To heal the sense of sin and the various resulting maladies, we practice yoga to help increase *shanti* (peace) and *shakti* (vitality). Peace helps us develop wisdom, the ability to see situations objectively. Vitality gives us the energy to practice compassion, serving others. When wisdom and compassion arise within a human being he is said to be healed. He has overcome the root illusion that he is a feeble, pitiful sinner and has claimed his birthright as a divine soul who is expressing the love and respect of his creator.

To reduce suffering, or to even just feel a little bit better, we engage in yoga *sadhana* (practice). We first practice feeling good in our body; then we extend that feeling into the deeper reaches of ourselves, healing the discontentment and inferiority complex. And then, as the great yoga really begins, we extend the good feelings out into the world, into our lives of relationships and commitments. We generously love those with whom we are close, and we generously forgive others with whom we may experience conflict.

As we practice yoga in order to end suffering and live a life of wisdom and compassion, we find that the basic nature of the world does not change. The seasons still come and go, night and day still revolve, and sickness and death are still the lot of everyone. But the miracle, the real miracle, is that the drama of human life is seen within a grand context of spiritual beauty. It still hurts when you stub your toe or when a loved one falls ill or dies. Yet, somehow, in the very core of the soul, we know there exists a light of eternal love that constantly shines upon all. Yoga is a simple and accessible means of accessing this light in the most immediate of places—in the body, in the breath, in the mind. When the yoga of body, breath, and mind becomes firm, the suffering born of the illusion of separation from God ceases, and one can truly rest in peace.

YES INTERNATIONAL PUBLISHERS
Award-winning books for personal self-transformation

Prem Prakash
  Yoga American Style
  Universal Yoga: The Bhagavad Gita for Modern Times
  Three Paths of Devotion: Goddess, God, Guru
Justin O'Brien, Ph.D. (Swami Jaidev Bharati)
  Walking with a Himalayan Master: An American's Odyssey
  Superconscious Meditation
  A Meeting of Mystic Paths: Christianity and Yoga
  The Wellness Tree: Dynamic Six-Step Program for Optimal Wellness
  Running and Breathing
  Mirrors for Men: A Journal for Reflection
Linda Johnsen
  Kirtan: Chanting as a Spiritual Path (with Maggie Jacobus)
  The Living Goddess: Reclaiming the Tradition of the Mother of the Universe
  Daughters of the Goddess: The Women Saints of India
  A Thousand Suns: Designing Your Future with Vedic Astrology
Swami Veda Bharati
  The Light of Ten Thousand Suns
  Subtler than the Subtle: The Upanishad of the White Horse
Theresa King
  The Spiral Path: Explorations into Women's Spirituality
  The Divine Mosaic: Women's Images of the Sacred Other
Phil Nuernberger, Ph.D.
  The Warrior Sage: Life as Spirit
  Strong and Fearless: The Quest for Personal Power
Charles Bates
  Pigs Eat Wolves: Going into Partnership with your Dark Side
  Ransoming the Mind: Integration of Yoga and Modern Therapy
Swami Hariharananda Bharati
  The Laughing Swami: Teachings of Swami Hariharananda
Christin Lore Weber
  Circle of Mysteries: The Woman's Rosary Book
Ron Valle and Mary Mohs
  Opening to Dying and Grieving: A Sacred Journey
Alla Renee Bozarth
  Soulfire: Love Poems in Black and Gold
Gopala Krishna
  The Yogi: Portraits of Swami Vishnu-devananda
Cheryl Wall
  Mirrors for Women: A Journal for Reflection
Mary Pinney Erickson and Betty Kling
  Streams from the Sacred River: Women's Spiritual Wisdom

The quarterly journal of the Institute of the Himalayan Tradition: *Himalyan Path*